Assessing Technology Platforms for Global Health Engagement to Support Integration of Efforts Across Geographic Combatant Commands

PADMAJA VEDULA, TRUPTI BRAHMBHATT, JONATHAN TRAN, CHANDLER SACHS

Prepared for the Office of the Assistant Secretary of Defense for Health Affairs
Approved for public release; distribution unlimited

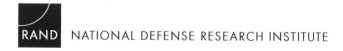

RAND NATIONAL DEFENSE RESEARCH INSTITUTE

For more information on this publication, visit **www.rand.org/t/RRA1357-3**.

About RAND

The RAND Corporation is a research organization that develops solutions to public policy challenges to help make communities throughout the world safer and more secure, healthier and more prosperous. RAND is nonprofit, nonpartisan, and committed to the public interest. To learn more about RAND, visit www.rand.org.

Research Integrity

Our mission to help improve policy and decisionmaking through research and analysis is enabled through our core values of quality and objectivity and our unwavering commitment to the highest level of integrity and ethical behavior. To help ensure our research and analysis are rigorous, objective, and nonpartisan, we subject our research publications to a robust and exacting quality-assurance process; avoid both the appearance and reality of financial and other conflicts of interest through staff training, project screening, and a policy of mandatory disclosure; and pursue transparency in our research engagements through our commitment to the open publication of our research findings and recommendations, disclosure of the source of funding of published research, and policies to ensure intellectual independence. For more information, visit www.rand.org/about/research-integrity.

RAND's publications do not necessarily reflect the opinions of its research clients and sponsors.

Published by the RAND Corporation, Santa Monica, Calif.
© 2023 RAND Corporation
RAND® is a registered trademark.

Library of Congress Cataloging-in-Publication Data is available for this publication.

ISBN: 978-1-9774-1092-4

Cover: *Marleah Cabano/U.S. Air Force.*

About This Report

The U.S. Department of Defense (DoD) has been conducting global health engagement (GHE) worldwide for nearly 125 years. Initially, such engagements were developed to protect service members from infectious diseases that were local to the areas they were deployed. DoD has since invested in the research and monitoring of infectious diseases in partner nations and, according to some key reports, has been instrumental in the prevention and treatment of, and the development of vaccines and other countermeasures for, various infectious diseases. Today, GHE is an instrument of strategic engagements, employing "forward medical diplomacy" for DoD to execute the U.S. National Defense Strategy. GHE is an integral part of the cooperation efforts of DoD and geographic combatant commands (GCCs) with partner nations and provides support in training and preparing their military and civilian health systems.

A capabilities-based assessment (CBA) of GHE, funded by the Deputy Assistant Secretary of Defense for Health Readiness Policy and Oversight and conducted using the DOTmLPF-P framework, was completed in July 2018.[1] Although the CBA affirmed the importance of GHE, it also identified numerous gaps and proposed 15 recommendations to improve the effectiveness and efficiency of GHE activities in contributing to GCC Theater Campaign Plan (TCP) objectives. The recommendations were compiled in a DOTmLPF-P Change Recommendation (DCR), which was endorsed in a Joint Requirements Oversight Council Memorandum. RAND's National Defense Research Institute was tasked by the Office of the Assistant Secretary of Defense for Health Affairs (OASD[HA]) to conduct research for the following DCR actions related to GHE:

- funding mechanisms and authorities
- education and training
- technology and process requirements to support (1) the life cycle of activities and assessments—from planning to evaluation—and (2) the information- and knowledge-sharing needs.

The purpose of this research was to develop a set of strategic recommendations for DoD, OASD(HA), and the GCCs to support the GHE community and increase the effectiveness, efficiency, and visibility of its engagements. The research was conducted as three parallel studies for the DCR actions related to the three categories mentioned above.

This report is one of three reports documenting the research for the three study categories.[2] This report focuses on the technology and process requirements to support (1) the life cycle of activities and assessments—from planning to evaluation—and (2) the information- and knowledge-sharing needs of the GHE community. We assessed platforms and solutions to support GHE activities and training (Actions 7 and 9 of the

---

[1] DOTmLPF-P stands for Doctrine, Organization, Training, materiel, Leadership and education, Personnel, Facilities, and Policy.

[2] The two other reports in this series are Jefferson P. Marquis, Trupti Brahmbhatt, Aaron Clark-Ginsberg, Victoria M. Smith, and David E. Thaler, *Educating and Training the Department of Defense Workforce for Global Health Engagement to Support the Geographic Combatant Commands*, RAND Corporation, RR-A1357-1, 2023; and Beth Grill, Trupti Brahmbhatt, Pauline Moore, Jennifer D. P. Moroney, and Chandler Sachs, *Funding Global Health Engagement to Support the Geographic Combatant Commands*, RAND Corporation, RR-A1357-2, 2023.

DCR).[3] We describe the methodological approaches, findings, and recommendations related to the assessment of technology platforms and intelligence- and knowledge-sharing needs of the GHE practitioners and GHE leadership. Finally, we present a set of recommendations for GHE leadership in OASD(HA) and the GCCs to implement policies for better integration of information and to support better collaboration and intelligence-sharing among GHE practitioners.

RAND National Security Research Division

This research was sponsored by the Office of the Assistant Secretary of Defense for Health Affairs and conducted within the Personnel, Readiness, and Health Program of the RAND National Security Research Division (NSRD), which operates the National Defense Research Institute (NDRI), a federally funded research and development center sponsored by the Office of the Secretary of Defense, the Joint Staff, the Unified Combat-ant Commands, the Navy, the Marine Corps, the defense agencies, and the defense intelligence enterprise. For more information on the RAND Personnel, Readiness, and Health Program, see www.rand.org/nsrd/prh or contact the director (contact information is provided on the webpage).

Acknowledgments

We are grateful to the Office of the Assistant Secretary of Defense for Health Affairs, David Smith, Terry Rauch, and J. Christopher Daniel, our project monitor, for sponsoring this study, and for Dr. Daniel's invaluable guidance and support. We would also like to thank the Office of Deputy Assistant Secretary of Defense for Health Readiness Policy and Oversight and the Center for Global Health Engagement for their invaluable insights. We are indebted to the global GHE community across GCCs, component commands, services, and other offices for sharing their expertise, opinions, and time with us. Additionally, we wish to thank GHE information technology infrastructure program managers, project leads, and their teams for their time, patience, and willingness to share information, demonstrate platforms, and address questions on requirements and road maps on multiple occasions.

Finally, we wish to thank many RAND colleagues who offered insights on the study and expertise on platforms used by GHE, the intelligence community, and the security cooperation organizations. We are grateful for our research reviewers: Molly McIntosh, Daniel Ginsberg, and John Bordeaux. We would also like to thank Danielle Smith, Holly Johnson, and Karin Suede for their assistance in preparing these reports, tracking down research papers, note-taking, and setting up classified meetings.

---

[3]   DCR Action 7, under the Training category, states the need to "[c]onduct a feasibility study on the development of a Joint GHE 'Intellipedia' site . . . for the GHE community. The site should include . . . best practices, templates, frameworks, and links to the training modules on GHE activities." DCR Action 9, under the Materiel category, states the need to

> [c]onduct a technology survey to identify potential government off-the-shelf (e.g., Joint Civil Information Management System) and commercial off-the-shelf solutions that satisfy the requirement to systematically identify, collect, synthesize, analyze, and report data relating to the environment to enable accurate problem articulation and planning. Solutions should work towards being compatible and aligning with current online information management systems used for GHE. (Paul Selva, Vice Chairman of the Joint Chiefs of Staff, "DOTmLPF-P Change Recommendation for Global Health Engagement," memorandum, JROCM 008-19, February 25, 2019, Attachment A, p. 3, Not available to the general public)

Summary

Global health engagement (GHE) is one of the strategic tools of the U.S. Department of Defense (DoD) for executing the U.S. National Defense Strategy.[4] GHE is an integral part of the cooperation efforts of DoD with partner nations and provides support in training and preparing their military and civilian health systems. GHE helps build and sustain partner health capacity, as well as partner trust and stability. This helps create interoperability with partners to ensure the protection of deployed U.S. forces and provide medical readiness opportunities. Additionally, partner capacity-building helps create a joint effort, in collaboration with the U.S. interagency, in combating global health threats. GHE activities leverage DoD capabilities to execute a broad range of functions, including force health protection; foreign humanitarian assistance; foreign disaster relief; nuclear, chemical, and biological defense; infectious disease response; and other stability and security cooperation operations (Figure S.1).[5] These activities encompass a wide spectrum of engagements—military-to-military, military-to-civilian, and multilateral—and support joint missions of humanitarian aid and disaster response, deterrence, access and presence, counterterrorism, and homeland defense.[6] The importance of these activities has been particularly noticeable during the global response to the coronavirus disease 2019 (COVID-19) pandemic. GHE activities within the geographic combatant commands (GCCs) form a critical part of the U.S. government's global security cooperation apparatus and stability operations. GHE activities also enable the building of bilateral and multilateral relationships and interoperability that help support U.S. interests and security objectives.

Global health engagements and activities require extensive planning, funding, and resource allocation within the GCCs and component commands. For a continuously growing breadth of GHE and the need to support joint exercises with partner military and civilian medical professionals for partner capacity-building, GHE also requires the support of a robust information technology (IT) infrastructure. The IT infrastructure should be able to support various functions, both at the operational and tactical levels—military services, GCCs, and component commands—and at the policy development, planning, and program evaluation levels—including multiple Offices of the Secretary of Defense and the Joint Chiefs of Staff. GHE IT infrastructure consists of, and requires, platforms to broadly support (1) funding and activity tracking, (2) education and training of personnel and partner resources, (3) measurement, monitoring, and assessment of GHE activities for sustainment and medical readiness, (4) future planning and synchronization (Theater Campaign Plan [TCP] and resource allocation), (5) data analytics and reporting capabilities, and (6) collaboration and knowledge-sharing.

One of the strategic requirements of GHE and DoD decisionmakers, as described in Chapter 3 of this report, is to have the ability to create a common operating picture (COP) for GHE within the combatant commands and DoD. To support this requirement and other more-operational needs, the IT infrastructure should include:

- platforms that provide processes and capabilities to seamlessly integrate engagement data across GCCs
- access to current and historical data

---

[4] U.S. Southern Command, "Global Health Engagement Strengthens Partnerships," January 6, 2020.

[5] Department of Defense Instruction 2000.30, *Global Health Engagement (GHE) Activities*, U.S. Department of Defense, July 12, 2017.

[6] Joint Publication 3-39, *Foreign Humanitarian Assistance*, Joint Chiefs of Staff, May 14, 2019.

FIGURE S.1

Conceptual Framework for the Spectrum of DoD GHE Activities

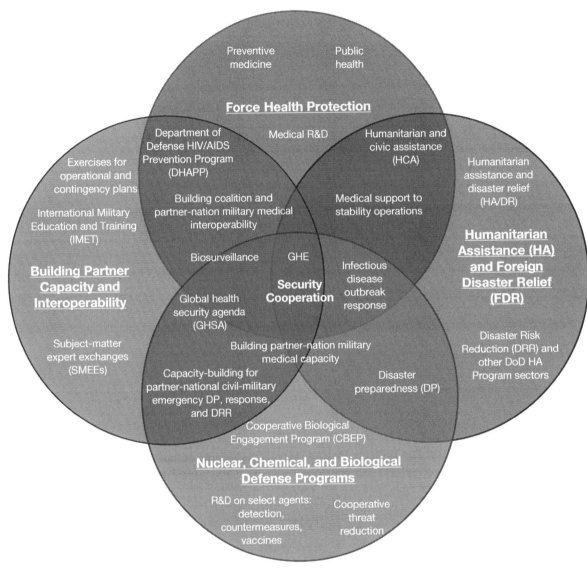

SOURCES: Adapted from Uniformed Services University, "Department of Defense Global Health Engagement," briefing, undated, Not available to the general public; and Department of Defense Instruction 2000.30, 2017, p. 4.

NOTE: R&D = research and development.

- tools for planning, funding, recording, and tracking GHE activities across the GCCs
- tools for reporting and analytics, and collaboration.[7]

A GHE capabilities-based assessment (CBA) was funded by the Deputy Assistant Secretary of Defense for Health Readiness Policy and Oversight and conducted using the DOTmLPF-P[8] framework.[9] Completed in July 2018, the CBA affirmed the importance of GHE capabilities in contributing to GCC TCP objectives and in "adding significant value to civilian-led global health efforts."[10] The CBA also identified numerous GHE capability gaps, including (1) the lack of availability of technology platforms and related policies that support the planning, capturing, tracking, monitoring, reporting, analyzing, and evaluation of the funding and execution of GHE activities and (2) insufficient understanding of how to engage the intelligence community and other relevant communities in support of GHE, along with a lack of information integration and knowledge exchange of DoD global health activities with civilian agencies and nongovernmental organizations. The CBA resulted in 15 recommendations to increase the effectiveness and efficiency of GHE activities in supporting GCC TCP objectives. The recommendations were compiled in a DCR and endorsed in a Joint Requirements Oversight Council Memorandum.[11]

The RAND National Defense Research Institute was tasked by the Office of the Assistant Secretary of Defense for Health Affairs (OASD[HA]) to conduct research for the DCR actions related to (1) GHE funding mechanisms and authorities, (2) education and training, and (3) technology and process requirements to enhance GHE capabilities, from the planning phase to the evaluation of activities, and to support information- and knowledge-sharing needs. The research was conducted as three parallel studies for the DCR actions related to the three categories mentioned above.[12] This report focuses on technology platforms and solutions to support GHE activities and training (Actions 7 and 9 of the DCR). Action 7, under the Training category, states the need to "[c]onduct a feasibility study on the development of a Joint GHE 'Intellipedia'[13] site . . . for the GHE community. The site should include . . . best practices, templates, frameworks, and links to the training modules on GHE activities." Action 9, under the Materiel category, states the need to

> [c]onduct a technology survey to identify potential government off-the-shelf (e.g., Joint Civil Information Management System) and commercial off-the-shelf solutions that satisfy the requirement to systematically identify, collect, synthesize, analyze, and report data relating to the environment to enable accurate prob-

---

[7] DoD, *Global Health Engagement (GHE) Capabilities-Based Assessment (CBA) Study*, July 23, 2018, Not available to the general public; and SME discussions.

[8] DOTmLPF-P stands for Doctrine, Organization, Training, material, Leadership and education, Personnel, Facilities, and Policy.

[9] Chairman of the Joint Chiefs of Staff Instruction 5123.01H, *Charter of the Joint Requirements Oversight Council (JROC) and Implementation of the Joint Capabilities Integration and Development System (JCIDS)*, Joint Chiefs of Staff, August 31, 2018.

[10] DoD, 2018.

[11] Selva, 2019, Attachment A.

[12] The two other reports in this series are Jefferson P. Marquis, Trupti Brahmbhatt, Aaron Clark-Ginsberg, Victoria M. Smith, and David E. Thaler, *Educating and Training the Department of Defense Workforce for Global Health Engagement to Support the Geographic Combatant Commands*, RAND Corporation, RR-A1357-1, 2023; and Beth Grill, Trupti Brahmbhatt, Pauline Moore, Jennifer D. P. Moroney, and Chandler Sachs, *Funding Global Health Engagement to Support the Geographic Combatant Commands*, RAND Corporation, RR-A1357-2, 2023.

[13] Intellipedia is a collaborative information-sharing tool for the intelligence community. Based on the concept of Wikipedia, it allows the creation of pages by topic, related metadata, and collaborative edits. For the intelligence community, it is available at all levels of classification (Gregory F. Treverton, *New Tools for Collaboration: The Experience of the U.S. Intelligence Community*, Center for Strategic and International Studies, January 2016.

lem articulation and planning. Solutions should work towards being compatible and aligning with current online information management systems used for GHE.[14]

Study Objectives and Approach

Our team conducted research related to these actions as two separate tasks to identify the stakeholders, program offices, and relevant supporting technologies and platforms for each action. We then sought to understand the requirements (the information needs) and the capabilities of the technology platforms that would support the planning and execution of activities, as well as assessment, monitoring, and evaluation (AM&E) approaches. We also sought to understand the gaps related to policy and processes, platform capabilities, and access of information for collaboration, decisionmaking, and analytics.

We addressed two main research questions (and several subquestions) based on the two technology-related DCR actions, as follows.

Assessment of Technology Platforms

What are the technology infrastructure requirements of GHE planners and practitioners, both at the GCCs and component commands and within the Office of the Secretary of Defense (OSD), to support the planning, execution, and AM&E of GHE activities? To address this question, we sought to answer the following:

- How are the current systems used? How do these systems align with the funding authorities and activities related to GHE?
- What requirements are being met by the current systems?
- What are the gaps in capability needs, bottlenecks, policy and process gaps, and interoperability and collaboration issues?
- What types of platforms, interfaces, processes, and policies would help alleviate these issues and provide a better picture to the decisionmakers?

Feasibility Study on the Development of a Joint GHE Intellipedia

How would the development of a joint GHE Intellipedia-like site improve collaboration and information-sharing among the GHE community? To address this question, we sought to answer the following:

- How would the GHE community benefit from the information shared on this site (in addition to the IT platforms already in place)?
- What features or tools could be offered by GHE Intellipedia that would be different from any other collaboration tools, such as dashboards, data visualization interfaces, and chatrooms?

One of the issues that the GHE community sought to address is the lack of integrated and comprehensive data and a COP of all the GHE activities in various GCCs and their components. Hence, we could not base this research on any significant existing data on global health engagements. Therefore, our team carried out the research using multiple qualitative methods. Our research approach consisted of three overlapping steps. First, we conducted a literature review of documentation, articles, and previous RAND research related to GHE activities, funding sources, and stakeholders; the DoD directives, instructions, and guidance on GHE

---

[14] Selva, 2019, Attachment A, p. 3.

and software systems; the evolution of technology solutions to support GHE; systems in use by GHE practitioners; and technology solutions in the market, focusing particularly on cloud infrastructure and services and cloud service providers. Concurrently, we identified and had discussions with subject-matter experts—at the GCCs and component commands, OSD, and the Center for Global Health Engagement, as well as technology platform product owners, program managers, and technical leads—to document and analyze GHE technology platform requirements.[15] Finally, we assessed available and planned platforms based on their features, enhancements, support and maintenance, data integration, interoperability, and future road maps. These steps and the coding and content analysis methods are described in Chapter 1. Chapters 2 and 3 provide detailed analysis of the requirements and feature support of current platforms. In Chapter 4, we summarize the results of our analysis and offer detailed recommendations for how OSD and OASD(HA) could facilitate such an improvement. Table S.1 provides a brief overview of the findings and recommendations to improve the support for GHE activities, practitioners, and planners by enhancing GHE IT infrastructure and the access to and capabilities of IT platforms. Additionally, we provide recommendations for future studies for deeper analysis into specific GHE capabilities, requirements, and GHE platform user insights.

---

[15] The discussions were conducted from the second half of 2020 to March 2021. Because of travel restrictions related to the COVID-19 pandemic, all discussions were conducted virtually. Platform demonstrations were also conducted virtually.

TABLE S.1

Findings and Recommendations

Research Question	Findings	Recommendations
Assessment of Technology Platforms		
• What are the technology infrastructure requirements of GHE planners and practitioners, both at the GCCs and at DoD and OSD to support planning, executing, and AM&E of GHE activities? – How are the current systems used? How do these align with the funding authorities and activities related to GHE? – What requirements are being met by the current systems? – What are the gaps in capability needs, bottlenecks, policy and process gaps, and interoperability and collaboration issues?	1. Current technology platforms do not support all GHE practitioners' requirements for capturing and tracking all activities. 2. Current platforms are not user-friendly, are not consistently maintained, and lack data standardization. 3. GHE practitioners have (1) limited access to historical data and information on current GHE engagements and (2) limited visibility into all GHE activities within one and across all areas of responsibility (AORs).	1. OASD(HA) should facilitate the creation of a GHE Integrated Product Team (IPT) to provide GHE-specific platform requirements and acceptance criteria to system developers. 2. The GHE community should leverage existing platforms, with the IPT directing future enhancements, maintenance, and usability. 3. The GHE technology platform should provide different process workflows to support different funding and activity needs. 4. The platform should support future GHE funding structure with integrated, accessible, and discoverable historical data on planning and funding activities, as well as after-action reviews (AARs) across all GCCs.
– What types of platforms, interfaces, processes, and policies would help alleviate these issues and help provide a better picture to the decisionmakers?	4. The GHE community seeks an integrated (and, ideally, a single) platform that would help with data access and visibility across GCCs, interoperability, sharing lessons learned, and cost analysis. 5. Mandates and policies must support GHE practitioners by enabling better data capturing and verification practices. 6. Data analytics capabilities are needed to showcase the value of GHE to combatant commanders, the Joint Chiefs of Staff, DoD civilian leadership, and the U.S. Congress.	5. The platform should provide continuous data integration with AOR-specific "homegrown" systems used by the GHE community and support the import data captured in siloed, on-premises systems. 6. The platform should include data entry compliance and verification to ensure the completeness of ongoing and after-action updates of GHE activities. 7. The GHE IPT should continuously monitor and communicate data and verification policies with platform program management. 8. The GHE platform(s) should provide advanced data analytics capabilities that leverage integrated GHE data to enable reporting, forecasting, planning, and decisionmaking for GHE leadership.
Feasibility Study on Joint GHE Intellipedia		
• How would the development of a joint GHE Intellipedia-like site improve collaboration and information-sharing among the GHE community? – How would the GHE community benefit from the information shared on this site (in addition to the IT systems already in place)? – What features or tools could be offered by GHE Intellipedia that would be different from any other collaboration tools, such as dashboards, data visualization interfaces, and chatrooms?	7. The GHE community sees little value in a separate GHE Intellipedia site, despite Common Access Card (CAC) access, because of issues with maintenance and ease of use. 8. Information shared on previous GCC Intellipedia pages was not intelligence and has been of little use beyond the GCC. 9. GHE practitioners prefer to use an integrated platform that also supports collaborative tools.	9. Because there is no demand signal for a separate GHE Intellipedia, the GHE community should consider other integrated platform alternatives to facilitate collaboration and knowledge- and intelligence-sharing. 10. The GHE community should explore the integration of data from platforms capturing lessons learned, AARs, and information on other joint events.

Contents

Figures and Tables

Figures

Tables

CHAPTER 1

Introduction

The U.S. Department of Defense (DoD) has been conducting global health engagement (GHE) worldwide for nearly 125 years. Initially, such engagements were developed to protect service members from infectious diseases that were local to the areas they were deployed.[1] The U.S. Army's efforts to prevent virulent diseases from threatening the health of troops during the Spanish-American War is an early example of the military's health engagements for force health protection.[2] DoD has since invested in the research and monitoring of infectious diseases in partner nations and, according to some key reports, has been instrumental in the prevention and treatment of, and the development of vaccines and other countermeasures for, various infectious diseases: for example, support for research on and prevention of diseases during the construction of the Panama Canal.[3] Other historical examples of what is now considered GHE include DoD support for humanitarian assistance and disaster relief and assisting partner nations by augmenting and building their health capabilities and capacities, starting with the Medical Civil Action Programs for treatment of local populations during the Vietnam War.[4]

Today, GHE is an instrument of strategic engagements, employing "forward medical diplomacy" for DoD to execute the U.S. National Defense Strategy.[5] GHE is an integral part of the cooperation efforts of DoD and the geographic combatant commands (GCCs) with partner nations and provides support in training and preparing their military and civilian health systems. GHE helps build and sustain partner health capacity and partner trust and stability. This helps create interoperability with partners to ensure the protection of deployed U.S. forces. Additionally, partner capacity-building helps create a joint effort, in collaboration with the U.S. interagency, in combating global health threats. GHE activities leverage DoD capabilities to execute a broad range of functions, including force health protection; foreign humanitarian assistance; foreign disaster relief; nuclear, chemical, and biological defense; infectious disease response; and other stability and security cooperation operations (Figure 1.1).[6] These activities encompass a wide spectrum of engagements—military-to-military, military-to-civilian, and multilateral—and support joint missions of humanitarian

---

[1] DoD, Military Health System, "Global Health Engagement," webpage, undated.

[2] Kelly Ayotte, Julie Gerberding, and J. Stephen Morrison, *Ending the Cycle of Crisis and Complacency in U.S. Global Health Security. A Report of the CSIS Commission on Strengthening America's Health Security*, Center for Strategic and International Studies, November 2019.

[3] Bryce H. P. Mendez, Sara M. Tharakan, and Emily K. Lane, "Department of Defense Global Health Engagement," Congressional Research Service, IF11386, updated January 16, 2020.

[4] DoD, Military Health System, undated; and Michael W. Wissemann, "Great (Soft) Power Competition: US and Chinese Efforts in Global Health Engagement," *Parameters*, Vol. 51, No. 3, August 2021.

[5] Suzanne Leclerc-Madlala and Maysaa Alobaidi, "Sharpening Our Cultural Tools for Improved Global Health Engagement," *Joint Force Quarterly*, No. 82, July 2016; and U.S. Southern Command, "Global Health Engagement Strengthens Partnerships," January 6, 2020.

[6] Department of Defense Instruction 2000.30, *Global Health Engagement (GHE) Activities*, U.S. Department of Defense, July 12, 2017.

FIGURE 1.1

Conceptual Framework for the Spectrum of DoD GHE Activities

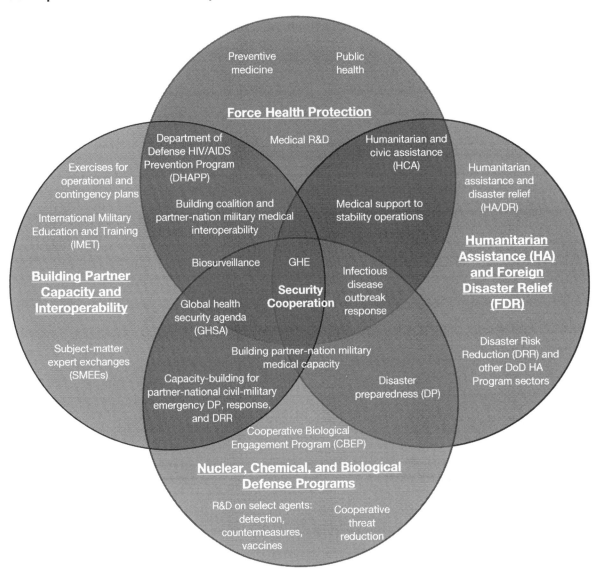

SOURCES: Adapted from Uniformed Services University, "Department of Defense Global Health Engagement," briefing, undated, Not available to the general public; and Department of Defense Instruction 2000.30, 2017, p. 4.

NOTE: R&D = research and development.

aid and disaster response, deterrence, access and presence, counterterrorism, and homeland defense.[7] The importance of these activities has been particularly noticeable during the past two years of global response to the coronavirus disease 2019 (COVID-19) pandemic. GHE activities within the GCCs form a critical part of the U.S. government's global security cooperation apparatus and stability operations. GHE activities also enable the building of bilateral and multilateral relationships and interoperability that help support U.S. interests and security objectives.

Global health engagements and activities require extensive planning, funding, and resource allocation within the GCCs and component commands. For a continuously growing breadth of GHE and the need to

---

[7] Joint Publication 3-29, *Foreign Humanitarian Assistance*, Joint Chiefs of Staff, May 14, 2019.

support joint exercises with partner military and civilian medical professionals for partner capacity-building, GHE also requires the support of a robust information technology (IT) infrastructure.[8] The IT infrastructure should be able to support various capabilities, both at the operational and tactical levels—military services, GCCs, and component commands—and at the policy development, planning, and program evaluation levels—including the Office of the Secretary of Defense (OSD), the Office of the Assistant Secretary of Defense for Health Affairs (OASD[HA]) , and the Joint Chiefs of Staff. Table 1.1 shows a list of capabilities that are required in GHE IT infrastructure and platforms.

To support these requirements and other more-operational needs, the IT infrastructure should include platforms that provide:

- processes and capabilities to seamlessly integrate engagement data across GCCs
- access to current and historical data
- tools for planning, funding, recording, and tracking GHE activities across the GCCs
- tools for reporting, analytics, and collaboration.[9]

A GHE capabilities-based assessment (CBA) was funded by the Deputy Assistant Secretary of Defense for Health Readiness Policy and Oversight and conducted using the DOTmLPF-P[10] framework.[11] Completed in July 2018, the CBA affirmed the importance of GHE capabilities in contributing to the accomplishment of GCC Theater Campaign Plan (TCP) objectives and in "adding significant value to civilian-led global health efforts."[12] The CBA also identified numerous GHE capability gaps, including (1) the lack of availability of technology platforms and related policies that support the planning, capturing, tracking, monitoring, reporting, analyzing, and evaluation of the funding and execution of GHE activities and (2) insufficient understanding of how to engage the intelligence community and other relevant communities in support of GHE,

TABLE 1.1

List of High-Level Capabilities Required in GHE IT Platform(s)

Capabilities	Office or Commands
Funding and activity tracking	GCCs, Component Commands, Other
Education and training of personnel and partner resources	GCCs, Component Commands
Measurement, monitoring, and assessment of GHE activities for sustainment and medical readiness	GCCs, OSD
Future planning and synchronization: TCP and resource allocation	GCCs
Data analytics and reporting	GCCs, OSD
Collaboration and knowledge sharing	GCCs
Common operating picture (COP)	GCC Surgeons General, OSD

---

[8] DoD, *Global Health Engagement (GHE) Capabilities-Based Assessment (CBA) Study*, July 23, 2018, Not available to the general public.

[9] DoD, 2018; and SME discussions.

[10] DOTmLPF-P stands for Doctrine, Organization, Training, material, Leadership and education, Personnel, Facilities, and Policy.

[11] Chairman of the Joint Chiefs of Staff Instruction 5123.01H, *Charter of the Joint Requirements Oversight Council (JROC) and Implementation of the Joint Capabilities Integration and Development System (JCIDS)*, Joint Chiefs of Staff, August 31, 2018.

[12] DoD, 2018.

along with a lack of information integration and knowledge exchange of DoD global health activities with civilian agencies and nongovernmental organizations (NGOs). The CBA resulted in 15 recommendations to increase the effectiveness and efficiency of GHE activities in supporting GCC TCP objectives. Those recommendations were compiled in a DOTmLPF-P Change Recommendation (DCR), which was endorsed in a Joint Requirements Oversight Council Memorandum.[13]

RAND National Defense Research Institute was tasked by OASD(HA) to conduct research for the DCR actions related to (1) GHE funding mechanisms and authorities, (2) education and training, and (3) technology and process requirements to enhance GHE capabilities, from the planning phase to the evaluation of activities, and to support the information- and knowledge-sharing needs. The research was conducted as three parallel efforts for the DCR actions related to the three categories mentioned above.[14] This report focuses on technology platforms and solutions to support GHE activities and training (Actions 7 and 9 of the DCR). Action 7, under the Training category, states the need to "[c]onduct a feasibility study on the development of a Joint GHE "Intellipedia"[15] site . . . for the GHE community. The site should include . . . best practices, templates, frameworks, and links to the training modules on GHE activities." Action 9, under the Materiel category, states the need to

> [c]onduct a technology survey to identify potential government off-the-shelf (e.g., Joint Civil Information Management System) and commercial off-the-shelf solutions that satisfy the requirement to systematically identify, collect, synthesize, analyze, and report data relating to the environment to enable accurate problem articulation and planning. Solutions should work towards being compatible and aligning with current online information management systems used for GHE.[16]

Methodology

Our team conducted research related to these actions to identify the stakeholders, program offices, and relevant supporting technologies and platforms for each action. We then sought to understand the requirements (the information needs) and the capabilities of the technology platforms that would support the planning and execution of activities, as well as assessment, monitoring, and evaluation (AM&E) approaches. We also worked to understand the gaps related to policy and processes, platform capabilities, and access of information for collaboration, decisionmaking, and analytics. Per consultation with our study monitor, we limited this study to evaluating DoD platforms only after we determined that either current platforms or those under development by DoD could be considered as feasible options.

---

[13] Paul Selva, Vice Chairman of the Joint Chiefs of Staff, "DOTmLPF-P Change Recommendation for Global Health Engagement," memorandum, JROCM 008-19, February 25, 2019, Attachment A, Not available to the general public.

[14] The two other reports in this series are Jefferson P. Marquis, Trupti Brahmbhatt, Aaron Clark-Ginsberg, Victoria M. Smith, and David E. Thaler, *Educating and Training the Department of Defense Workforce for Global Health Engagement to Support the Geographic Combatant Commands*, RAND Corporation, RR-A1357-1, 2023; and Beth Grill, Trupti Brahmbhatt, Pauline Moore, Jennifer D. P. Moroney, and Chandler Sachs, *Funding Global Health Engagement to Support the Geographic Combatant Commands*, RAND Corporation, RR-A1357-2, 2023.

[15] Intellipedia is a collaborative information-sharing tool for the intelligence community. Based on the concept of Wikipedia, it allows the creation of pages by topic, related metadata, and collaborative edits. For the intelligence community, it is available at all levels of classification (Gregory F. Treverton, *New Tools for Collaboration: The Experience of the U.S. Intelligence Community*, Center for Strategic and International Studies, January 2016.

[16] Selva, 2019, Attachment A, p. 3.

For studying the feasibility of implementing a GHE Intellipedia-like site, we sought to understand the requirements from stakeholders of a platform for collaboration, knowledge-sharing, and accessing GHE handbook, templates, and best practices. We also tried to understand the usability of such a site and the current knowledge-sharing bottlenecks that it may address.

We addressed two main research questions (and several subquestions) based on the two technology-related DCR actions, as follows.

Assessment of Technology Platforms

What are the technology infrastructure requirements of GHE planners and practitioners, both at the GCCs and at DoD and OSD, to support planning, executing, and AM&E of GHE activities? To address this question, we sought to answer the following:

- How are the current systems used? How do these systems align with the funding authorities and activities related to GHE?
- What requirements are being met by the current systems?
- What are the gaps in capability needs, bottlenecks, policy and process gaps, and interoperability and collaboration issues?
- What types of platforms, interfaces, processes, and policies would help alleviate these issues and provide a better picture to the decisionmakers?

Feasibility Study on the Development of a Joint GHE Intellipedia

How would the development of a joint GHE Intellipedia-like site improve collaboration and information-sharing among the GHE community? To address this question, we sought to answer the following:

- How would the GHE community benefit from the information shared on this site (in addition to the IT systems already in place)?
- What features or tools could be offered by GHE Intellipedia that would be different from any other collaboration tools, such as dashboards, data visualization interfaces, and chatrooms?

One of the issues that the GHE community sought to address is the lack of integrated and comprehensive data and a COP of all the activities in various GCCs and their components. Hence, we could not base this research on any significant existing data on global health engagements. Therefore, our team carried out the research using multiple qualitative methods. Our research approach consisted of three overlapping steps. First, we conducted a literature review of documentation, articles, and previous RAND research related to GHE activities, funding sources, and stakeholders; the evolution of technology solutions to support GHE; systems in use by GHE practitioners; and technology solutions in the market, focusing particularly on cloud infrastructure and services and cloud service providers. Concurrently, we identified and held discussions with GHE subject-matter experts (SMEs)—at the GCCs and component commands, OSD, and the Center for Global Health Engagement (CGHE), as well as technology platform product owners, program managers, and technical leads—to document and analyze GHE technology platform requirements.[17] The discussions were conducted using the discussion protocols listed in Appendix A. Appendix C lists the stakeholder SMEs and platform program offices with whom we had discussions. Finally, we assessed the available and planned

---

[17] The discussions were conducted from the second half of 2020 to March 2021. Because of travel restrictions related to the COVID-19 pandemic, all discussions were conducted virtually. Platform demonstrations were also conducted virtually.

platforms based on their features, enhancements, support and maintenance, data integration, interoperability, and future road maps. Using the platform requirements gathered to support GHE collaboration and knowledge-sharing needs, we compared the technological investment required to set up, maintain, and use a GHE Intellipedia-like site with the usability, SME interest, and benefits of having such a site to the larger GHE community. For the technology platform assessment, we first designed a high-level approach to address the research questions and visualize the possible outcomes and recommendations. The high-level approach was created to identify the key steps in the assessment process. Figure 1.2 illustrates the approach as a flowchart. The steps include selecting a methodology for the assessment, identifying the need to receive requirement inputs and feedback from both GHE practitioners and SMEs and platform program offices, researching the possible solutions (including a single GHE cloud-based platform), creating an evaluation framework, and the formulating recommendations.

Based on the high-level approach and industry methods to assess current and legacy systems, we formulated the research methodology as described earlier in this section. Figure 1.3 illustrates this methodology, composed of the frameworks for the three key steps: requirements analysis, evaluation, and recommendations.

Figure 1.4 illustrates the methodology for studying the feasibility of standing up a new joint GHE Intellipedia site, as described earlier in this section.

For both studies, we used two separate criteria developed according to GHE practitioner requirements and business needs (nontechnical) and the technical assessments of the platforms.[18] We weighted the criteria according to the importance of each requirement to stakeholders—both GHE practitioners and platform management (the number of stakeholder inputs for a certain requirement)—and according to whether a

FIGURE 1.2
GHE Technology Platform Assessment: High-Level Approach

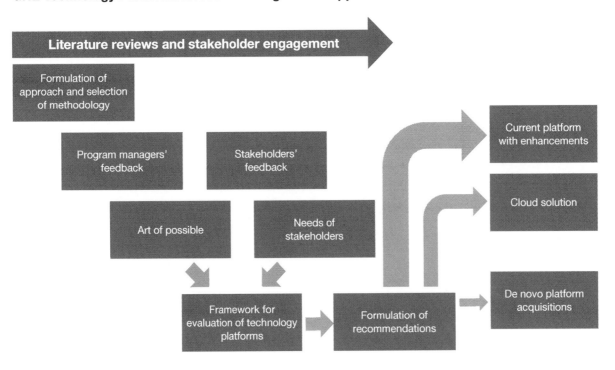

---

[18] For the feasibility study for a GHE "Intellipedia," the business (nontechnical) requirements, or *business value*, took precedence over the *technical value* (or quality) for two reasons: (1) the site would have been a new implementation and (2) technical value evaluation could not be completed because of the lack of business interest and lack of access to information on the current intelligence community Intelink and Intellipedia.

FIGURE 1.3

Methodology for Technology Platform Survey and Assessment

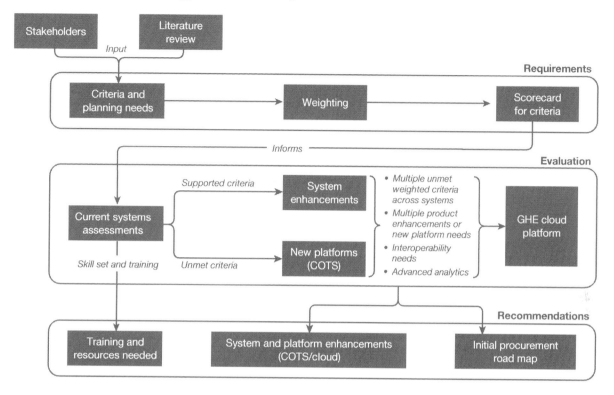

NOTE: COTS = commercial off-the-shelf.

FIGURE 1.4

Methodology for Intellipedia Feasibility Study

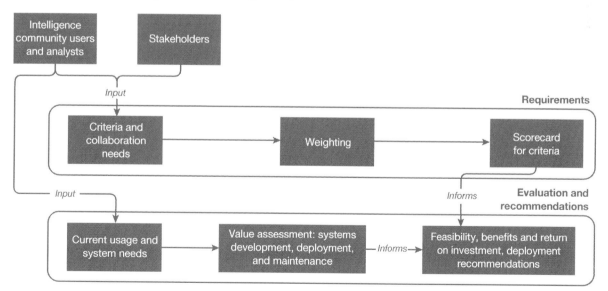

requirement is important to support the current GHE engagement scope or whether it is "nice to have." We describe this weighting further in Chapter 2. For technical assessment, the weighting was added according to the current usability and maintenance of the platform, future enhancements in development, and the future road map for feature support. Appendix A provides both frameworks for the coding and content analysis of GHE stakeholder inputs and requirements and for the technical system analysis based on the following criteria (Box 1.1), taking the key stakeholder requirements, as identified in Chapter 2, into consideration.[19]

We did a high-level assessment of business value using the inputs of stakeholders, experts, and reviews of previous RAND research. High-level assessments help in recognizing the platforms that are closest to meeting the requirements for or are currently used for tracking main GHE engagement data. This assessment was followed by the detailed assessment for weighting using the two coding and content analysis frameworks mentioned above (Appendix A).[20] Using a decisional matrix (as shown in Figure 1.5), also known as a chi-square chart,[21] to plot the platforms, we can assess the combined weight of technical and business criteria of the current platforms used by GHE, or the need for a new GHE platform, against each quadrant, as described in Table 1.2.

BOX 1.1
Derived Criteria for Platform Technical Quality Assessment

Organization and Management Strategy
- Vision: Which business objectives of the organization is the platform meant to support?
- Responsible organization: Organization responsible for the development and maintenance of the platform
- Structure: What are the supported organizational procedures, roles, and responsibilities?
- Management of GHE life-cycle funding: Which funding streams and activities are supported?
- Technological dependencies: Operating systems, data systems, and other platforms that the system is dependent on

System Features
- Program or system of record status
- Platform architecture: Technology configuration, cloud environment, size, software and hardware reliability
- Classification and access: At what classifications is the platform available, and what are the requirements for user access?
- Development and maintenance: Development methodologies used and ease of maintenance

System Analysis
- Adequacy and scalability: Does the platform meet the needs (performance); diffusion (across GCCs); platform portability
- Maturity: Improvements and new technologies (e.g., cloud based), investments in enhancements, upkeep (new releases)
- Interoperability: Capability of the platform to be integrated and supported by other platforms and technologies

User Experience
- Usability of the system: System complexity of user interface, documentation, performance

---

[19] Criteria are based on attributes from the following sources: Lerina Aversano and Maria Tortorella, "An Assessment Strategy for Identifying Legacy System Evolution Requirements in eBusiness Context," *Journal of Software Maintenance and Evolution Research and Practice*, Vol. 16, No. 4–5, July–October 2004; James Crotty and Ivan Horrocks, "Managing Legacy System Costs: A Case Study of a Meta-Assessment Model to Identify Solutions in a Large Financial Services Company," *Applied Computing and Informatics*, Vol. 13, No. 2, July 2017; and Jane Ransom, Ian Sommerville, and Ian Warren, "A Method for Assessing Legacy Systems for Evolution," *Proceedings of the Second Euromicro Conference on Software Maintenance and Reengineering*, 1998.

[20] Ransom, Jane, Ian Sommerville, and Ian Warren, 1998.

[21] Priyadarshi Tripathy and Kshirasagar Naik, *Software Evolution and Maintenance: A Practitioner's Approach*, Wiley, 2015, pp. 197–198.

FIGURE 1.5

Business Value and Technical Quality Decision Matrix

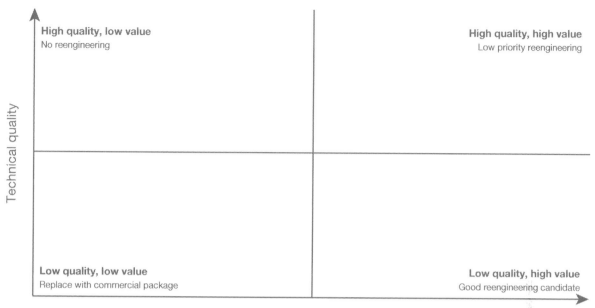

SOURCE: Adapted from Ransom, Sommerville, and Warren, 1998, p. 6.

TABLE 1.2

Interpretation of Matrix Assessment

Quadrant	Assessment	Notes
• Low business value • Low technical quality	• Replace with commercial package	• Need for very high investment in improvement; replacement with COTS solution preferable.
• Low business value • High technical quality	• No reengineering	• No enhancements or upgrades required. Gradually discontinue use of platform or integrate with more high-value platform.
• High business value • High technical quality	• Low priority reengineering	• Invest in continuous enhancements. "Should be actively evolved."[a]
• High business value • Low technical quality	• Good reengineering candidate	• Add enhancements to upgrade, or upgrade to a new platform.

SOURCES: Features information from Ransom, Sommerville, and Warren, 1998; and Robert C. Seacord, Daniel Plakosh, and Grace A. Lewis, *Modernizing Legacy Systems: Software Technologies, Engineering Processes, and Business Practices*, Addison-Wesley, 2003.

[a] Seacord, Plakosh, and Lewis, 2003, p. 30.

This decision matrix is generally used to perform a detailed analysis, primarily of legacy software platforms; however, it was still useful to apply to the platforms used by GHE to determine whether there is a need for continuous enhancements of some of these systems to support GHE requirements or for a new GHE platform specifically to support all GHE engagements across GCCs.[22] In Chapter 3, we plot the main platforms used by the GHE community for tracking engagements on the chi-square chart. Additionally, we illustrate this assessment in a stop-light chart.

---

[22] Some platforms used by GHE are relatively new and have only gone into production as recently as October 2020.

Research Limitations

One of the primary limitations that we faced was that our research was conducted entirely during the COVID-19 pandemic; hence, all interactions with SMEs and product teams were online, using Microsoft Teams conferences, telephone conversations, and document-sharing. SMEs and product teams were contacted via email, and the discussion protocols were sent prior to the discussions. Most of the technology product demonstrations were also online, in both classified and unclassified settings. We made several attempts to obtain read-only and/or view-only access to some technology products. However, because of firewalls and other issues related to the DoD Common Access Card (CAC), we could not obtain permission for such access. In lieu of this access, we used multiple online product demonstrations and product documentations. A DoD memorandum on "Software Development and Open-Source Software" reflects DoD's push toward an "Adopt, Buy, Create" approach to software platforms.[23] DoD is looking to "preferentially [adopt] existing government or OSS [open-source software] solutions before buying proprietary offerings."[24] Because we had already identified several DoD platforms used for GHE, in consultation with our study monitor, we did not evaluate COTS platforms.

For studying the feasibility of setting up GHE Intellipedia, we consulted with several experts (including GHE stakeholders and RAND experts) who use or have used the current Intellipedia site. RAND experts included those who access Intellipedia sites used by the intelligence community for research and analysis. Some GHE practitioners from GCCs who had set up Intellipedia sites or pages for collaboration also provided their inputs and evaluations with regard to their ease of use and maintainability. The ownership of Intelink (the host network for Intellipedia) and Intellipedia was initially set up with the Central Intelligence Agency, Defense Intelligence Agency (DIA), and the National Security Agency (NSA). NSA hosts and maintains the Intelink network as of today. Even after several attempts, we could not find any contacts at NSA or DIA for follow-up meetings. Hence, our assessment of Intellipedia and other Intelink tools and their usability and usefulness for the GHE community was done based on documentation, RAND expert knowledge, and inputs from GHE practitioners and stakeholders, including CGHE experts. This analysis is detailed in Chapters 2 and 3.

Organization of This Report

The organization of this report is based on the steps followed in our research, as illustrated in the methodology section. In Chapter 2, we document the analysis of our discussions with GHE stakeholders and former GHE practitioners across various GCCs, CGHE, and DoD leadership. We also document the key requirements that we derived for the GHE technology platforms and Intellipedia needs according to a literature review of open-source information, previous RAND reports, and stakeholder insights gathered during the discussions on the current systems being used, including support for GHE funding and activities, challenges and usability, unmet functionality needs, and preferred features in future GHE technology solutions. For the GHE Intellipedia study, we also determined the collaboration and knowledge- and intelligence-sharing needs (within and beyond the GHE community), as well as the usability requirements. These requirements

---

[23] John B. Sherman, U.S. Department of Defense Chief Information Officer, "Software Development and Open Source Software," memorandum for senior Pentagon leadership, Commandant of the Coast Guard, commanders of the combatant commands, and defense agency and DoD field activity directors, January 24, 2022, p. 3.

[24] Sherman, 2022, p. 3.

formed a part of the criteria for accessing the current IT platforms and possible future infrastructure, as described in the methodology section.

In Chapter 3, we document the analysis of various IT platforms and solutions used by the GHE community based on the discussions with the platform program manager(s) and project leads, system documentation and future road maps, and an assessment of requirements against enhancements of existing platforms or platforms in development for GHE and the security cooperation apparatus. We also document our analysis on the requirements and value of acquiring a "de novo" platform for GHE according to the functional and technical criteria, user requirements criteria, and decision matrix as described in this chapter.

Finally, in Chapter 4, we summarize the results of our analysis and present recommendations for increasing the effectiveness and interoperability of GHE IT platforms to support efficient execution of GHE activities across GCCs. We also recommend specific platforms that would support both the GHE practitioners and the GHE planners and leadership.

CHAPTER 2

Determining Information System Needs of GHE Stakeholders

GHE Information Platform Requirements

To analyze and understand GHE technology platform needs and compare them with the available platforms for the GHE community, we conducted discussions with both GHE stakeholders and the program management of current IT platforms (Appendix C). We held discussions with GHE SMEs at all GCCs and the U. S. Special Operations Command (SOCOM), component commands, relevant OSD offices, service GHE representatives, and CGHE. Additionally, we identified 14 platforms to evaluate the requirements for tasks related to both Action 7 and Action 9 of the CBA. These platforms are used by GHE practitioners to capture information on planning and funding activities, life cycles of activities, after-action reviews (AARs), lessons learned, monitoring and reporting, integrated views of various security cooperation programs and civil information, country information and medical intelligence, data engineering and analytics, and events involving partner-nation collaboration. We were able to engage with the management and project leads of 12 of these IT platforms. We held discussions with nine platform managers, received documentation from three, and had platform demonstration sessions with project teams of seven platforms. We also examined the future development road maps of some of the platforms, such as Socium, Medical Common Operating Picture (MedCOP), and Advana, described in detail in the next chapter and in Appendix D, by attending demonstration sessions and monthly product updates and by having follow-up discussions throughout their development from 2020 to 2022. Over the course of this study, we held discussions with 38 GHE practitioners and 22 information system program managers.

We then categorized the stakeholder inputs into the following framework: GHE platforms used, requirements, challenges, and preferred features, focusing particularly on the support for planning, funding, and executing GHE activities. For the GHE Intellipedia-like site, requirements focused on the usability, SME interest, benefits and return on investment, and technical complexity and maintainability of sites on Intellipedia.

To summarize, various platforms are used by GHE stakeholders to capture engagements and activities where global health engagements are conducted or have an important medical component (such as exercises). The GCCs, through their service components, conduct global health engagements. Because GHE is an umbrella term, activities that are considered GHE are spread across authorities in the armed forces; therefore, tracking these activities is also spread across various IT platforms, both by authority and by area of responsibility (AOR).

The COVID-19 pandemic increased the use of collaborative platforms as the spread of the pandemic, directives from DoD limiting travel, and required quarantine periods (both in the United States and abroad) limited the ability to hold in-person events. Collaboration has, however, been mostly for internal teams that use virtual meeting software (Microsoft Teams, Blue Jeans, ZoomGov, etc.), while other services, such as the All Partners Access Network (APAN), allow for collaboration and document-sharing with foreign partners.

GHE stakeholders find many of the platforms used by GHE limited in terms of feature support, user-friendliness, and maintainability. For example, despite options for capturing information on both DoD-wide and GCC-specific "homegrown" platforms, many GHE practitioners still use spreadsheets and text files to capture information, which are generally stored on local document servers (SharePoint) or personal devices. This makes GHE activity data siloed and inaccessible for future reference, reporting, or analytics. Hence, any future attempts for data integration across platforms should not be limited to platform data imports or automated updates between platforms but will have to consider importing data captured in local servers and computers, taking the issues of data standards and validations into consideration. We identified the following requirement criteria for a future GHE platform based on the stakeholder inputs on current platforms: challenges, preferred features, and nice-to-have features.

The following GHE platform requirements received almost equal weighting from stakeholders, except for the final two, which have been categorized as "nice to have":

- **User-friendly.** The platform should be easy to create and update funding request and activity data with supporting verification and workflows.
- **Consistently maintained.** The platform should have consistent maintenance, enhancements, and product support.
- **Able to capture all activities, all "medical things."** Many of the current GHE and security cooperation platforms (both DoD-wide and GCC-specific) offer support for specific funding authorities or a specific type of activities. GCCs also have difficulty in getting insight from various service components into other engagements that may be service-funded or that are rolled up in an exercise from other types of funding. This results in the use of multiple systems, siloed data streams, and limited view into all activities within one and across all GCCs. An integrated platform that supports multiple funding streams, with one-way or two-way data flow with existing GHE platforms, would allow GHE practitioners to capture and access information on all historical and ongoing activities.
- **Include standardized data.** Current GHE activity data are captured in siloed platforms or applications, are related to specific funding streams, and do not have common and complete data elements or semantics. For integration of data across platforms in the future, this is a significant bottleneck that would need to be addressed.
- **Enforce policies related to mandatory use and data verification.** This is not only required for data compliance but also vital for insights into requirements, funding, and collaboration across GCCs and for reporting, analyzing, and planning future activities. This would also be important to align Lines of Effort in the GCC's TCP with outcomes for creating a COP.
- **Provide accessible, integrated data from prior engagements** (AARs, measures of performance and effectiveness, templates of previous successful proposals, and site-based policies and doctrines).
- **Provide visibility over all the activities within one and across all AORs.**
- **Support integrated analytics capabilities for a COP of GHE activities.** Platforms should support data collections, collection of metrics, analysis of raw data, and future artificial intelligence (AI) capabilities for advanced analytics and planning support.

"When you look at everyday engagements (going in to do exercises, clinics, meetings, conferences, etc.), I think there's a big difference between what we were doing and what the IT systems were capturing. Again, if you're a senior leader in D.C. trying to make decisions about the value of GHE, I don't think your dashboard is mature enough to understand the extent of it, the range of activities ongoing, and where the gaps are either in countries or capability sets."
SOURCE: GHE SME discussion, March 2, 2021.

- Ideally, there should be a single platform for GHE for data, interoperability, exchange of information, lessons learned, and cost analysis (nice-to-have).
- Platform should incorporate data captured in handheld and stand-alone devices, which are not on the network (nice-to-have).[1]

Table 2.1 presents a business value scorecard for platforms used by GHE or platforms being developed for security cooperation and GHE, based on the stakeholder inputs and requirements.[2] In Chapter 3, we describe these platforms. Additional platforms used by the GHE community are discussed in Appendix D. The scores are calculated as the number of positive stakeholder inputs divided by the number of stakeholder inputs, recoded to adjust the scores for "homegrown" platforms or platforms that are used only by certain GCCs or GHE practitioners.

TABLE 2.1

Business Value Scorecard of Platforms Based on Requirements Criteria

Requirements	Platforms Used by GHE Practitioners for Engagement Data				
	G-TSCMIS	CFR	OHASIS	Socium[a]	MedCOP[a]
User friendly	0.11	0.33	0.44	0.77	1
Consistently maintained	0.11	0.33	0.55	1	1
Captures all activities, all "medical things"	0	0	0.22	0.55	0.66
Includes standardized data	0.11	0.33	0.44	1	1
Enforces policies related to mandatory use and data verification	0	0.33	0.22	1	0.66
Accessible integrated data from prior engagements	0.55	0.33	1[b]	1	0
Visibility over all the activities within one and across all AORs	0.11	0.11	0.11	0.66	0
Integrated analytics capabilities for a COP of GHE activities (AI support)	0	0	0	0.66	1
Ideally, a single platform for GHE[c]	0	0	0	0.22	0
Incorporate data captured in hand-held/ stand-alone devices which are not on network[c]	0	0	0	0	0
Total	0.99	1.76	2.98	6.86	5.32

NOTE: G-TSCMIS = Global-Theater Security Cooperation Management Information System; CFR = Concept and Funding Request; OHASIS = Overseas Humanitarian Assistance Shared Information System. CFR is a GCC-specific platform used by U.S. European Command (EUCOM), U.S. Africa Command (AFRICOM) and U.S. Central Command (CENTCOM; which uses and maintains an older version of CFR). Information from stakeholder discussion on November 6, 2020.

[a] Stakeholder also spoke for potential future capabilities. MedCOP discussions were conducted with a smaller stakeholder community due to it being a relatively newer platform for GHE.

[b] Prior funding requests only.

[c] Nice to have.

---

[1] The last two requirements are identified as nice-to-have because a single platform to capture all GHE activities would result in redundant workload on GHE practitioners when the activity is tied to a larger theater engagement, funding, or exercise. Many GHE activities are funded as part of larger GCC or component command efforts. For incorporation of data captured in handheld devices on the field into an integrated GHE platform, we could not assess the current capabilities and potential for future enhancements because of platform management having other features with higher priorities in the pipeline. A future study in this area might be useful.

[2] Table 2.1 lists only the platforms that directly support many of the GHE activity planning, funding, and tracking needs across GCCs.

GHE Intellipedia: Requirements and Usability

For the feasibility study of setting up an Intellipedia site, the following requirements were identified by the stakeholders for collaboration and knowledge-sharing:

- a single site or repository for all applicable policies and doctrine: DoD Instruction 2000.30, DoD Instruction 2205.02, force health protection, foreign disaster relief, etc.
- access to previously approved proposals to give practitioners an insight into the proposals that are likely to be funded and how to format and submit them
- resources on colors of money (funding sources)
- GHE- and GCC-specific playbooks and best practices
- lessons learned, including integration of information captured in current systems, such as the Joint Lessons Learned Information System (JLLIS) and Geographic Information System (GIS)
- military-civil and military-to-military chatrooms
- workspace where entities can share in bulletin board format, storage spaces, etc.
- site or platform should be easy to access and easy to use
- site or platform should be consistently maintained.

Many GHE stakeholders added certain caveats to setting up a GHE Intellipedia site, as follows:

- Previous attempts at creating and maintaining pages and sites on the intelligence community's Intellipedia on Intelink (discussed in Chapter 3) by GHE practitioners at different GCCs were not successful because the sites were not used for intelligence-sharing across the GHE community. The sites were generally used for event notices and sharing documentation for specific exercises.
- Previous Intellipedia pages and sites were not maintained consistently. Today, the sites are not in use, and information on these sites is obsolete, with broken links. GHE Intellipedia might have similar maintenance issues if the demand signal is low or if it would not be easy to access, use, and maintain.
- GHE practitioners prefer an integrated platform that provides support for the aforementioned requirements, including chatrooms, enabling easy access for collaboration.

> "We have Intellipedia [pages] attached to everything DoD [has] created in the last ten years and they're all empty. You need a forcing function for DoD to use one singular program. We move systems every two to three years, [and we] need [a] whole new set of log-ins."
> SOURCE: GHE SME discussion, February 25, 2021.

In the next chapter, we provide the technical and feature support analysis of the current GHE platforms and develop a technical quality scorecard of existing platforms that currently support or might support GHE requirements with further enhancements. We then map the business values (as presented in Table 2.1) and the technical quality to determine the need, if any, for a GHE de novo platform development or to propose existing or in-development platforms with high business value and high technical quality as candidates for the future integrated GHE platform.

CHAPTER 3

Analysis of Current and Proposed Information Systems for GHE

Using the technology survey methodology and system analysis framework (Appendix A), we assessed 12 technology platforms used by the GHE community and assessed the "met" and "unmet" criteria as identified in Chapter 1: i.e., the required product features and enhancements to support GHE activities, interoperability and data integration needs to support the stakeholder requirement of visibility of current and past activities across GCCs, requirement of a COP for decisionmakers and planners, ease of use, maturity of platforms, maintenance and enhancement support, and program of record status. We also looked at the unmet criteria along with stakeholder inputs on an "ideal single GHE platform" (as described in Chapter 2) to assess the need for a new COTS platform or a single GHE cloud-based platform.

We performed a literature review of documentation and articles related to GHE activities and funding sources; related RAND research on the evolution of technology solutions to support GHE; the DoD directives, instructions, and guidance on GHE and software systems; and current systems used by GHE practitioners. We also performed a high-level assessment of technology solutions in the market, focusing particularly on cloud infrastructure and services and cloud service providers. Based on these two efforts, we developed an initial set of driving factors for a new COTS cloud-based platform for GHE (Table 3.1). We used these factors to develop the infrastructure requirements of a new GHE platform.

TABLE 3.1

Driving Factors for New Cloud-Based Platform

Driving Factors	Benefits of Cloud Services	Outcome
Literature and current trends review reveals transition to cloud-based services for data-intensive IT solutions in both GHE and DoD. Examples of ongoing and proposed implementations: • Socium • Knowledge Management Concept • Defense Information Systems Agency "Authorized DoD Cloud Service Catalogue," 2018 • Joint Enterprise Defense Infrastructure (JEDI 2.0)	• Security and compliance[a] (Defense Security Cooperation Agency [DSCA] Cloud, Amazon Web Services [AWS] GovCloud) • Database and data warehousing services (AWS Redshift, AWS RDS) • Data analytics (AWS Textract, AWS SageMaker, Electronic Medical Records, etc.) • Cost and pricing (Kathryn Connor, Ian P. Cook, Isaac R. Porche III, and Daniel Gonzales, *Cost Considerations in Cloud Computing*, RAND Corporation, PE-113-A, 2014) • IT support	Based on requirements provided by stakeholders and program managers in discussions, we identified the following initial infrastructure needs for a GHE platform: • GHE platform should leverage cloud-based deployment and maintenance, scaling and load-balancing and software-as-a-service (SaaS) and platform-as-a-service (PaaS) offerings of a cloud environment. • Platform should leverage data storage, warehousing, data scrubbing, engineering, and analytics support of a cloud environment. • GHE platform should use current DoD-certified cloud service providers for security and multilevel classification needs and deployments.

[a] Based on DoD Cloud Computing Security guidelines.

A DoD memorandum on "Software Development and Open-Source Software" reflects DoD's push toward an "Adopt, Buy, Create" approach to software platforms.[1] DoD is looking to "preferentially [adopt] existing government or OSS [open-source software] solutions before buying proprietary offerings, and only creating new non-commercial software when no off-the-shelf solutions are adequate."[2] Our approach, as described in Chapter 1, is to assess the current platforms used by GHE using the criteria identified in Table 1.1, taking into account any unmet criteria to create a scorecard for the technical quality of the platform(s), similar to the scorecard for business value created in Chapter 2. In the event that all platforms have low scores, which is equivalent to multiple unmet criteria, and fall outside of the "High Quality, High Value" quadrant in the decision matrix (Figure 1.5 and Table 1.2), we would create a recommended road map for a new GHE cloud-based platform. In order to make this determination, we provide the technical quality assessment of GHE platforms in this section for both Action 7 and Action 9 of the DCR. We then provide the final evaluation of the platforms using the four quadrants in the decision matrix. For Intellipedia feasibility (Action 7), we use the user demand signal as the primary driving factor, along with an assessment of comparable platforms to determine the benefits or drawbacks of investing in a new GHE Intellipedia site.

In the following sections, we provide a detailed analysis of the primary technology platforms used by the GHE community. We first present the results of a technology assessment of the platforms associated with Action 9 of the DCR. This includes systems that are responsible for the tracking and managing of requests and funding of GHE activities, such as G-TSCMIS, CFR, OHASIS, Socium, and MedCOP. We then focus on platforms associated with Action 7 of the DCR: the feasibility of developing an Intellipedia-like capability for GHE. For this analysis, we address the Intellipedia (Intelink), JLLIS, and MedCOP platforms.

GHE Mission Data Systems

As part of the technology assessment, we initially conducted research and discussions for all technology platforms used by GHE shown in Appendix C. Concentrating on Action 9 of our study, we focused on the systems that track and manage GHE activities, which includes G-TSCMIS, CFR, OHASIS, Socium, and MedCOP. Additional platforms used by the GHE community are discussed in Appendix D. Table 3.2 provides a detailed technical assessment of current platforms by assigning each feature or component identified in Box 1.1 with a value for full, partial, or no support (recoded as 1, 0.5, and 0, respectively).[3]

Table 3.3 provides an overall high-level assessment of the selected platforms against our stakeholder requirements.

Here, we provide some historical context, and justification, for the high-level assessment in Table 3.3. In terms of the platform requirements analysis and technical baselining, we assess that G-TSCMIS provides a useful example and lessons learned for subsequent platforms. OHASIS and CFR are examples of systems actively used by the GHE community that are effective tools despite having limited funding support and use cases and despite being limited to specific GCCs. Socium and MedCOP are examples of the direction in which security cooperation systems are heading: flexible platforms with many use cases that are being developed to support multiple workflows, even though they are not matured platforms when compared to CFR or OHASIS. Socium and MedCOP both have development and maintenance teams and make use of agile "sprint" development cycles to implement iterative enhancements to the respective platforms. However, it is

---

[1] Sherman, 2022, p. 3.

[2] Sherman, 2022, p. 3.

[3] Aversano and Tortorella, 2004; Crotty, and Horrocks, 2017; and Ransom, Sommerville, and Warren, 1998.

TABLE 3.2

Technical Quality Scorecard of Platforms Based on Weighted Criteria

Technical Features	Platforms Used by GHE Practitioners for Engagement Data				
	G-TSCMIS	CFR	OHASIS	Socium	MedCOP[a]
Management of GHE life-cycle funding: Which funding streams and activities are supported?	1	1	1	0.5	0
Technological dependencies: Operating systems, data systems, other platforms that the system is dependent on[b]	0	0	0	0.5	0.5
Program or system of record status	1	1	1	1	0
Platform architecture: Technology configuration, cloud environment (scalability), size, software and hardware reliability	0	0	0	1	1
Development and maintenance: Development methodologies used and ease of maintenance	0	1	0	1	1
Adequacy and scalability: Does the platform meet the needs (performance); diffusion (across GCCs); platform portability	0	0	0	1	1
Maturity: Improvements and new technologies (e.g., cloud based), investments in enhancements, upkeep (new releases)	0	1	0	1	1
Interoperability: Capability of the platform to be integrated and supported by other platforms and technologies	0	1	0	0.5	0
Usability of the system: System complexity of user interface, documentation, performance	0	1	0	1	1
Total	2	6	2	7.5	5.5

[a] Taking some of the potential future capabilities into consideration.

[b] Is the platform fully integrated with its technological dependencies (other platforms and data sources)?

TABLE 3.3

Comparison of Platforms Based on GHE Requirements

Requirement	G-TSCMIS	CFR	OHASIS	Socium	MedCOP
User-friendly	X	✓	O	O	✓
Consistently maintained	X	✓	✓	✓	✓
GHE-focused "all medical things"	X	O	✓	O	O
Program of record	✓	✓	✓	✓	O
Activity life-cycle management	X	O	✓	O	X
Enforce policies related to mandatory use	✓	✓	✓	✓	O
Data entry verification to ensure completeness (i.e., data standardization)	X	✓	✓	✓	O
Provide ability to pair activities with long-term planning and strategy	X	✓	X	O	X
Provide visibility over all activity types across all AORs	X	X	X	✓	O
Support integrated analytic capabilities	X	X	X	O	✓
Single platform	X	X	X	O	X

NOTE: Green (✓) = requirements supported; yellow (O) = requirements not completely supported or still in development; red (X) = requirements not supported.

a challenge for the GHE community to communicate their priorities and requirements to the developers of the platforms, who support a large number of security cooperation stakeholders.

In subsequent sections, we provide a more-detailed analysis of the platforms mentioned above. We then present our assessment of the feasibility and need for a GHE Intellipedia site. We also present alternative tools that could meet the collaboration requirements stated in Chapter 2. We close this chapter with a decisional matrix based on the scorecards in Tables 2.1 and 3.2 for platforms for GHE activities. In Chapter 4, we present detailed findings and recommendations for the two study tasks for Action 7 and Action 9 of the GHE DCR.

Global-Theater Security Cooperation Management Information System

In December 2008, the G-TSCMIS acquisition strategy was added to the Deputy Secretary of Defense memorandum for G-TSCMIS for the establishment of a new development program. This was in response to a requirement originally identified by SOCOM for a management information system that would provide a whole-of-government view of the security cooperation COP. DoD Directive 5132.03, *DoD Policy and Responsibilities Relating to Security Cooperation*, mandated the use of the G-TSCMIS as the system for security cooperation activities.[4] This was followed by DoD Instruction 5132.14, *Assessment, Monitoring, and Evaluation Policy for the Security Cooperation Enterprise*, on January 13, 2017.[5]

Historically, the GHE and security cooperation activities were tracked separately by combatant commands on such systems as Service Integration Management (SIAM) by U.S. Indo-Pacific Command (INDOPACOM), Theater Engagement Planning Management Information System (TEPMIS) by EUCOM, and TSCMIS by U.S. Southern Command (SOUTHCOM).[6] The fiscal year (FY) 2017 National Defense Authorization Act provided several stipulations for the consolidation of authorities and instructions on the improvement of management and oversight of DoD security cooperation policy and programs. All legacy security cooperation management information from the activity records previously stored on the Army Global Outlook System and GCC TSCMISs were then migrated to G-TSCMIS.[7]

As a result, G-TSCMIS was designed to be "the overall collaborative tool and authoritative data source for DoD security cooperation assessment, planning, execution, monitoring, and evaluation."[8] G-TSCMIS facilitated the tracking of resources for and visibility into security cooperation activities and their statutes across DoD components. This provided insight into resources used for operation and maintenance and promoted the exchange of best practices. G-TSCMIS also integrated the project data funded by Overseas Humanitarian, Disaster, and Civil Aid (OHDACA) from the OHASIS.

---

[4] DoD Directive 5132.03, *DoD Policy and Responsibilities Relating to Security Cooperation*, U.S. Department of Defense, December 29, 2016.

[5] DoD Instruction 5132.14, *Assessment, Monitoring, and Evaluation Policy for the Security Cooperation Enterprise*, U.S. Department of Defense, January 13, 2017

[6] Jefferson P. Marquis, Richard E. Darilek, Jasen J. Castillo, Cathryn Quantic Thurston, Anny Wong, Cynthia Huger, Andrea Mejia, Jennifer D. P. Moroney, Brian Nichiporuk, and Brett Steele, *Assessing the Value of U.S. Army International Activities*, RAND Corporation, MG-329-A, 2006; and Jefferson P. Marquis, David E. Thaler, S. Rebecca Zimmerman, Megan Stewart, and Jeremy Boback, *The Global-Theater Security Cooperation Management Information System: Assessment and Implications for Strategic Users*, RAND Corporation, RR-1680-OSD, 2016, Not available to the general public.

[7] Angela O'Mahony, Ilana Blum, Gabriela Armenta, Nicholas E. Burger, Joshua Mendelsohn, Michael J. McNerney, Steven W. Popper, Jefferson P. Marquis, and Thomas S. Szayna, *Assessing, Monitoring, and Evaluating Army Security Cooperation: A Framework for Implementation*, RAND Corporation, RR-2165-A, 2018; and Walter L. Perry, Stuart Johnson, Stephanie Pezard, Gillian S. Oak, David Stebbins, and Chaoling Feng, *Defense Institution Building: An Assessment*, RAND Corporation, RR-1176-OSD, 2016.

[8] Joint Publication 3-20, *Security Cooperation*, Joint Chiefs of Staff, May 23, 2017, p. xii.

As noted by our engagement with GHE stakeholders, there were several disadvantages to G-TSCMIS. First, the G-TSCMIS contract included the initial development but no guaranteed funds for maintenance and future development. G-TSCMIS also lacked the enforcement of standardized data entry and analytic capabilities. Stakeholders often mentioned difficulty collecting data on activities from different offices and ensuring no duplication. Although the use of G-TSCMIS was mandated to access funding for security cooperation activities, data would often be entered after funding had been rewarded or after the activity was complete. Data were also sometimes added to meet compliance requirements, and most records had the bare minimum information required for creating entries in G-TSCMIS. It was also challenging for GHE planners to review activities because of the lack of information provided at different phases of the activity.[9] The CFR system refers to this process as an *activity life-cycle management system*. This frequently resulted in an incomplete view of security cooperation activities and contributed to the inability of the GHE community to showcase their engagements and the importance of GHE to DoD stakeholders.

Concept and Funding Request

The CFR platform was developed in 2011 and is the program of record at EUCOM, currently the primary user of CFR. AFRICOM and CENTCOM are also using the platform (CENTCOM owns an earlier version of the platform that it maintains separately from the version used by EUCOM and AFRICOM). CFR has been made available for use by any combatant command or organization, but it is not an integrated, globally accessible platform. Each instantiation of CFR is distinct and tailored to the organization; however, it is used in all cases to track information about a given engagement, such as funding amounts, approval, the command lawyer review, J5 strategy and policy review, and after-action assessments. It is also mandatory for securing Section 312 funding to support a proposed short-term military-to-military engagement in both EUCOM and AFRICOM, which accounts for approximately 60 percent to 70 percent of all GHE funding in the respective combatant commands. EUCOM currently allocates funds to support a team of three IT specialists who are dedicated to the maintenance of the system.[10]

Despite sharing many of the engagement tracking capabilities of systems such as G-TSCMIS and Socium, stakeholders in EUCOM have emphasized that CFR plays a larger role in the funding approval process. Within EUCOM, those who wish to be funded by Section 312 EUCOM funding, Section 164 authority funding for U.S travel, Section 1251 events, Section 321 events, or Institute for Security Governance Civil-Military Emergency Preparedness Program events are required to submit a request for funding through CFR. This results in the first key difference between CFR and other tracking systems: CFR tracks both successful and unsuccessful proposals. Approximately two months prior to the allocation of funds (typically near the end of April), CFR is locked, packaged, and distributed to the EUCOM country desk offices. Each proposal is then weighed against the respective country SMARTObjectives[11] and subsequent milestones, resulting in an assigned numerical Strength of Coordination value and feedback from the desk offices.[12] A high Strength of Coordination value indicates the proposal is tied more closely to the country objectives and likelihood for funding. This activity life-cycle management review process is a key argument for the continued use of CFR. An example of an activity life cycle for Section 312 events is provided in Figure 3.1.

---

[9] Stakeholder discussions conducted in 2020 and 2021.

[10] Perry et al., 2016.

[11] SMART stands for Specific, Measurable, Achievable, Realistic, and Time-bound.

[12] Michael J. McNerney, Jefferson P. Marquis, S. Rebecca Zimmerman, and Ariel Klein, *SMART Security Cooperation Objectives: Improving DoD Planning and Guidance*, RAND Corporation, RR-1430-OSD, 2016.

FIGURE 3.1

Example Section 312 Activity Life Cycle

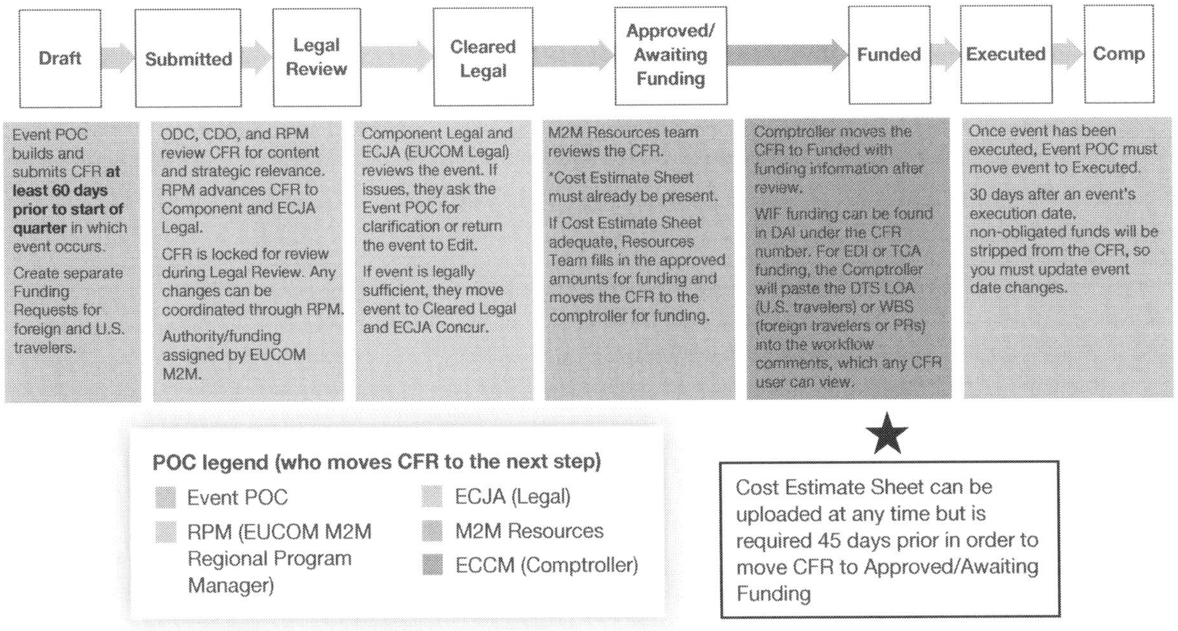

SOURCE: Adapted from U.S. European Command J5/8 Security Cooperation and Partnering Division, *M2M and Concept & Funding Request (CFR) User Guide*, May 20, 2020, p. 2.

We evaluated CFR as a potential platform to understand the platform's capacity to scale, support enhancements, and support other funding streams for a larger GHE community. GHE stakeholders have noted significant disadvantages to CFR. The first is the lack of a centralized CFR database. Each instantiation of CFR is distinct and only houses data for the respective GCC. This poses a challenge when attempting to view security cooperation activities across organizations. CFR is also focused on Section 312 funding and has no plans to expand capabilities to other funding sources. The data from CFR typically are exported and merged with other information systems to achieve a wholistic view of security cooperation.

Associated EUCOM CFR Systems

EUCOM makes use of several other systems in conjunction with CFR. These include SASPlan (Strategy for Active Security Plan), which outlines each country's SMARTObjectives and milestones; Significant Security Cooperation Initiative (SSCI) Portal;[13] Conference Registration System (CRS), which is used to register for upcoming conferences and events; and the Technology Service Corporation Record Exchange (TREX). TREX is a system that is used by EUCOM to take inventory of all GHE activities and events within a country across different IT platforms. EUCOM stakeholders have stated the short-term goal of integrating Socium and OHASIS data with CFR using TREX for a wholistic view of security cooperation within a country.

---

[13] According to the Defense Security Cooperation Agency's Institute of Security Governance,

> DoD established a Significant Security Cooperation Initiative (SSCI)-centric planning and resourcing process. SSCI-centric planning requires Combatant Commands to generate partnership assessments, Initiative Design Documents (IDD), and discrete proposals to obtain funding and authorization to train-and-equip our partners. Fully integrating ICB [institutional capacity-building] considerations at the beginning stages of this planning cycle and across authorities will help ensure that partner institutional shortfalls and the ability and will to address them are considered, generating more realistic objectives within country plans." (Defense Security Cooperation Agency, Institute of Security Governance, "Institutional Capacity Building: An Essential Component of Full Spectrum Capability Development," January 2021)

Overseas Humanitarian Shared Information System

OHASIS is the system of record and the primary source of data for tracking OHDACA funding and has become the primary source of data on current and historical DoD humanitarian assistance activities. OHASIS includes four of the five OHDACA programs (it does not include foreign disaster response). OHASIS provides a system for DSCA to manage the OHDACA project proposal process and for the combatant commands to track the execution of approved activities. Planners and program managers at the combatant commands document estimated costs for program proposals and include estimated obligation and commitment rates. Although OHASIS includes a tab for recording resources, program managers rarely provide information on disbursement of funds for a particular activity. DoD officials noted that OHASIS is not used for financial management.[14]

GHE stakeholders have noted that although OHASIS occasionally is not user-friendly, it is a robust system that effectively tracks and manages humanitarian assistance activities. They noted two primary issues: (1) support for only one type of funding and (2) a lack of data validation, resulting in empty records with little information. Similar to CFR, the scope of OHASIS is limited to only OHDACA funding, and the data typically are exported and merged with other information systems to achieve a wholistic view of security cooperation. There are no plans for OHASIS to expand capability to other funding sources. There are active discussions between OHASIS and Socium developers to automate the data pipeline from OHASIS to Socium.

Socium

In FY 2020, DSCA coordinated with the security cooperation apparatus to deploy a new application as the replacement to the G-TSCMIS application. DSCA deployed the Socium application as part of the G-TSCMIS program in September 2020.[15] Socium is a DoD system of record and is a cloud-based activity and work-flow management tool. Socium addresses the requirement for a platform that "provides a Department-wide technology capability to facilitate and integrate planning, budgeting, collaboration, program design, assessment, monitoring, evaluation, and reporting in support of all U.S. security cooperation activities."[16] Socium is available for users across all DoD entities, including military departments, combat support agencies, and GCCs, requiring only a CAC. The activities the user can perform in Socium depend on the roles and authorities selected and approved within the SAAR form. All users have the ability to view the data within Socium, and the different user roles and permissions are provided in Table 3.4. As part of supporting all U.S. security cooperation activities, the full Socium requirements include tracking and management of 44 funding

> "DSCA was given the responsibility to replace G-TSCMIS primarily because the community was not using the system. That is indicative of the proliferation of homegrown systems across the CCMDs [combatant commands]. G-TSCMIS wasn't adequate in that it wasn't meeting their needs in terms of actioning activity from its birth to its death. They had just been sending their homegrown data to G-TSCMIS in order to meet the requirement."
> SOURCE: GHE platform requirements owner discussion, November 20, 2022.

---

[14] Beth Grill, Michael J. McNerney, Jeremy Boback, Renanah Miles, Cynthia C. Clapp-Wincek, and David E. Thaler, *Follow the Money: Promoting Greater Transparency in Department of Defense Security Cooperation Reporting*, RAND Corporation, RR-2039-OSD, 2017.

[15] Socium is considered to be a part of the larger G-TSCMIS program that earlier consisted of only the G-TSCMIS application.

[16] Defense Security Cooperation Agency, *Fiscal Year 2022 President's Budget: Operation and Maintenance, Defense-Wide*, May 2021b, p. 6.

TABLE 3.4

Socium User Roles

User Role	Permissions
Analyst	A user can view all available data, upload relevant documents, provide comments, and build new report templates. This user can also participate in AAR.
Strategic Planner	A user can create/edit data in the Strategic Planning to align/develop strategic roles/ goals/ objectives across multiple levels. This data would not be entered prior to the start of an activity. This user can also enter assessment data and participate in AAR.
Activity Planner	A user can create/edit data in the Planning phase to start creating activities that align to strategic roles/goals/objectives. This user submits concepts and proposals for approval. This user can also enter assessment and monitoring data for activities and participate in AAR.
Implementing Agency Manager	A user from the military department or defense agency responsible for the execution of military assistance programs. The user can create/edit data in the Planning phase to review feasibility of activities and create/update data in the Execution phase. This user can also enter monitoring data for activities and participate in AAR.
Financial Integration Manager	A user can create/edit data in the planning and execution phase as it relates to financial data. This user can also participate in AAR.
Contributor	Any Socium user can be assigned individually by other users with the appropriate permissions to contribute to data fields that parallel the inviter's permissions. This user has the ability to create and edit data when invited to do so.
AM&E Manager	A user can perform assessment, monitoring, and evaluations (AM&E) of strategic objectives and activities. Creates/edits and approves relevant AM&E data in the in the Strategic Planning, Planning, Execution, and Evaluation phases.
Reviewer	A user can approve or reject proposed activities and adds comments to explain decision for respective organization.
Organization Data Manager	A user performs quality assurance (QA) and quality control duties (QC) relative to security cooperation data entered within their respective organization. This includes creating, editing, and deleting data throughout the Strategic Planning, Planning, Execution, and Evaluation phases. Limit fifteen (15) per organization.
Socium Administrator	A user responsible for updating workflows and account management for respective organization. Limit five (5) per organization.

SOURCE: Features information from Defense Security Cooperation Agency, "DSCA Socium SAAR Guide," provided to the authors by Socium Program Management, December 2020b, Not available to the general public.

authorities, provided in Table 3.5. In support of these different funding authorities, part of Socium's value proposition is the consolidation of activity data across IT systems.

Socium begun full development in early 2020, transitioning to three-week sprint development cycles. Since then, Socium is a full replacement of the G-TSCMIS system and all its capabilities on both the Secret Internet Protocol Router (SIPR) and Non-classified Internet Protocol Router (NIPR) networks. The funding sources supported by Socium are noted in Table 3.5.[17] In late 2020, the NIPR Socium platform was available for use, and a one-way data transfer from G-TSCMIS was proceeding. More recently, the Socium development team has implemented a replacement for the SIPR G-TSCMIS system as well. As a result, Socium is available on both NIPR and SIPR networks. As of this writing, Socium is developing a workflow for long-term and strategic planning, synchronization of unclassified and classified data, improvements to initiative workflows, and AM&E capabilities (shown in Figure 4.2 from Socium).[18]

---

[17] Socium was originally released as a minimally viable product in 2020 (Defense Security Cooperation Agency, "Socium— Building a Security Cooperation Management System Overview," briefing, 2020a, Not available to the general public).

[18] Socium Program Management, "Socium Monthly Demonstrations," Defense Security Cooperation Agency, December 2020 to January 2022.

TABLE 3.5
Socium Funding Authorities

Title 10, Chapter 16	Title 10, Other	Title 22	Temporary	Other
• 311	• 401	• FMS	• FY08 1233 CSF	• Title 50
• 312	• 402	• FMF[a]	• FY08 1234 Lift & Sustain	• 3711
• 321	• 404	• IMET[a]	• FY08 1234 ASFF	• 3712
• 322[a]	• 407	• PKO	• FY15 1206 Human	• 3713
• 333[a]	• 116[a]	• EDA	Rights Training	• Title 14
• 341[a]	• 2557	• DoD Drawdown	• FY15 1236 Counter ISIL	• 195
• 342	• 2561		• FY15 ERI	
• 343	• Other military-to-military		• FY16 USAI	
• 344			• FY16 EETI	
• 345[a]			• FY16 MSI	
• 346				
• 347				
• 348				
• 349				
• 350				

SOURCE: Features information from Defense Security Cooperation Agency, 2020a.

NOTE: ASFF = Afghan Security Forces Fund; CSF = Coalition Support Fund; EDA = Economic Development Administration; EETI = Eastern European Training Initiative; ERI = European Reassurance Initiative; FMF = Foreign Military Financing; FMS = Foreign Military Sales; IMET = International Military Education and Training; ISIL = Islamic State in Iraq and the Levant; MSI = Maritime Security Initiative; PKO = peacekeeping operations; USAI = Ukraine Security Assistance Initiative.

[a] Indicates that this authority is a priority for the Minimally Viable Product (MVP) released on September 30, 2020. For all authorities not included in the Socium MVP, a "generic activity workflow" capability (replicating the G-TSCMIS functionality) will be included.

In discussions with the DSCA Directorate of Information Management & Technology and the Socium development team, we received a road map of systems with plans to integrate historical data into Socium. These data are not exclusively related to GHE but instead include all security cooperation activities. These systems are visualized in Figure 3.2. The color of the system indicates the status of the data transfer as of February 2021, and the arrow indicates the direction of the data transfer. GIS reference data and humanitarian assistance data integration with the World Bank and U.S. Agency for International Development is also planned for FY 2023. The vision is to

> "enhance Socium's capability to maintain comprehensive, accessible information that enhances oversight and data-driven decision-making capability for strategic users and to allow leaders to align SC [security cooperation] resources to the National Defense Strategy, Theater Campaign Plans, and Integrated Country Strategies."[19]

Key User Committee

The Socium Key User Committee was put in place to reinforce the collaborative development approach by engaging with the user community within each organization. The Key User Committee organizations are listed in Box 3.1. In addition, the Socium development team hosts ongoing monthly demonstrations of the platform that are open to any stakeholders and potential users. These monthly demonstrations are an opportunity to showcase new capabilities and features and to receive feedback and questions from the community. Early Socium stakeholders, adopters, and users also have access to the Socium Test environment, which mimics the production environment with the same roles, permissions, and responsibilities the user has in the Socium application.[20] This continuous engagement with stakeholders allows the Socium team to (1) intro-

---

[19] Defense Security Cooperation Agency, *Department of Defense Fiscal Year (FY) 2022 Budget Estimates: Research, Development, Test & Evaluation, Defense-Wide*, May 2021a, p. 16.

[20] Socium Program Management, December 2020.

FIGURE 3.2
Socium Integration Roadmap

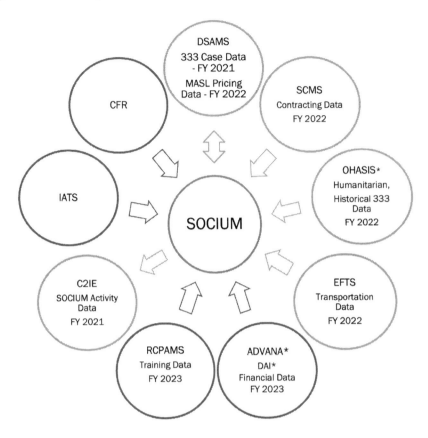

SOURCE: Reproduced from Defense Security Cooperation Agency IT Program Management, "Socium System Interfaces," February 2021, Not available to the general public.
NOTE: C2IE = Command and Control Information Exchange; DSAMS = Defense Security Assistance Management System; EFTS = Enterprise Freight Tracking System; IATS = Integrated Automated Travel System; RCPAMS = Regional Center Persons/Activity Management System; SCMS = Security Cooperation Management Suite.

duce new features as priorities, (2) fix issues identified, and (3) improve workflow development (using the agile development process), thereby mitigating the possibility of larger design issues being found after a new release.

Activity Life-Cycle Management

In addition to replicating the capabilities of G-TSCMIS, Socium has made several improvements, including capabilities to function as an activity life-cycle management system for all stages of an engagement. This feature allows the user to provide updates to an engagement over the course of an activity, including the strategic concept, activity concept, GCC concept review, and DSCA concept review. Activity life-cycle management can take place on any of the funding sources, including the Generic Activity Workflow, which is a default workflow for activities that do not fall into the specific workflows supported by Socium. When comparing the activity life-cycle management between Socium and CFR, it is clear CFR provides more intermediary stages and opportunities for users to submit or update data.[21] Socium, however, is designed to support all funding streams and engagements and iterative improvements to the life-cycle management process.

---

[21] Socium Program Management, December 2020 to January 2022.

BOX 3.1
Socium Key User Committee

Executive Departments and Staff
- DoD
- U.S. Department of State
- Joint Chiefs of Staff
- DoD agencies
- DSCA
- Defense Threat Reduction Agency
- GCCs
- AFRICOM
- CENTCOM
- EUCOM
- INDOPACOM
- U.S. Northern Command
- U.S. Southern Command

Military branches
- U.S. Army
- U.S. Navy
- U.S. Marine Corps
- U.S. Air Force
- U.S. Coast Guard
- U.S. National Guard Bureau
- Functional combatant commands
- U.S. Cyber Command
- U.S. Transportation Command

Geographic Information System

Socium-GIS is built on the commercial Environmental Systems Research Institute (ESRI) GIS capability and provides a visual interpretation of spatial and geographic data captured in Socium to enhance the user's analysis of security cooperation activities. The ESRI GIS infrastructure allows for automation of data analysis and workflows. As of January 2022, Socium has a NIPR GIS capability; the SIPR implementation is still in development.[22] All authorized Socium users will automatically receive access to Socium's Enhanced GIS.

Medical Common Operating Picture

The Defense Health Agency (DHA) Joint Operational Medicine Information System (JOMIS) program office has sponsored the development of the MedCOP platform. MedCOP supports the need for a complete command and control and situational awareness capability of all the DoD medical activities, assets, and programs across GCCs and other missions worldwide.[23] The JOMIS program office is responsible for "health information technology capabilities to meet existing and emerging operational medicine requirements" and

---

[22] Socium Program Management, December 2020 to January 2022.

[23] Betsy DeSitter and Max Ramirez, "MedCOP: A Step Towards Purple," *Medical Leader*, blog, October 22, 2020.

manages and maintains several medical technology platforms used by combatant commanders.[24] These systems include decisionmaking tools for health surveillance and for managing medical operations and services that provide analysis and visualization capabilities.

MedCOP began development in mid-2020. As of this writing, MedCOP is not a system or program of record; however, it resides as an application on the Automated Information Discovery Environment (AIDE) operating system,[25] which is a SOCOM and Joint Special Operations Command system of record. According to the MedCOP program development team, funding has been secured for MedCOP development through 2023. Although the initial focus was to replace existing JOMIS systems, including Medical Situational Awareness in Theater (MSAT), Medical Command and Control (MedC2), and Medical Situational Awareness (MedSA), GHE stakeholders have communicated interest in using MedCOP analytics and visualization capabilities for GHE activities and have stated a need for a one-way data transfer (both historical and real-time) from existing GHE tracking systems to MedCOP.[26] As of the writing of this report, discussions of the necessary requirements between GHE stakeholders and MedCOP were ongoing, and there were plans to implement GHE requirements iteratively. In addition to GHE activity data, real-time hospital and airport data are provided via Shoreland Travax.[27] There is a backlog requirement to integrate National Center for Medical Intelligence (NCMI) and Armed Forces Health Surveillance Branch data as well. The AIDE and MedCOP systems also use an agile software development process with a two-week development sprint timeline.

The AIDE operating system has additional applications that may be of use to GHE planners and practitioners. AIDE Drive is a file management system that also has file-sharing capabilities. ARES provides GIS capabilities and acts as the mapping application, allowing for real-time tracking of units and platforms in a battlespace. CEREBRO is a social media collaboration tool with community of interest, discussion board, and chat capabilities. Lastly, MedReports is used to integrate MedCOP with the previously mentioned applications. The AIDE platform (including MedCOP) is hosted on the DHA Amazon Web Services GovCloud, is available on both NIPR and SIPR networks, and is CAC and Public Key Infrastructure enabled, respectively.

MedCOP has several benefits, including an active development team, a robust analytic capability infrastructure (AIDE), and several collaborative tools, which we will emphasize in the next section. However, discussions with the development team as of January 2022 revealed that integration between MedCOP and GHE-related data sets remains a low priority. This is primarily due to a lack of explicit requirements put forward by the GHE community.

Collaboration Systems

As part of Action 7 of our study, we were tasked with assessing the feasibility of implementing a GHE Intellipedia-like site. The intention of a GHE Intellipedia is to provide the GHE community with a collabora-

---

[24] Deployed systems include AHLTA-Theater, Theater Medical Information Program (TMIP)-Composite Health Care System Cache, TMIP-Joint (TMIP-J), Theater Medical Data Store (TMDS), Deployed Tele-Radiology System/Theater Image Repository, Maritime Medical Modules, Medical Situational Awareness in Theater (MSAT), Defense Medical Logistics Standard Support Customer Assistance Module, U.S. Transportation Command Regulating and Command and Control Evacuation System (TRAC2ES), and Travax (Defense Healthcare Management Systems, "Joint Operational Medicine Information Systems" fact sheet, July 2020).

[25] Discussion with Program Support for JOMIS and MedCOP, April 2021; Novetta, "AIDE: Automated Information Discovery Environment," fact sheet, September 22, 2021.

[26] Of the existing GHE systems, Socium, OHASIS, and CFR have been mentioned explicitly by the MedCOP development team.

[27] Shoreland Travax, homepage, undated.

tive tool to share and disseminate information across GCCs and DoD. In this section, we discuss the Intelink-Intellipedia tool, and we focus on the feasibility and challenges of developing a comparable wiki tool. We also discuss the broader suite of Intelink collaboration tools provided on the SIPR network (shown in Figure 3.4). In addition to Intelink, we propose an alternative suite of tools provided by MedCOP that offers comparable capabilities (also shown in Figure 3.3).

Intelink

Intelink is a secure network set up for the U.S. intelligence community that has different installations for different levels of classifications. Intellipedia refers to a specific installation of wikis on Intelink used by the intelligence community for online information- and file-sharing and collaboration. Intellipedia is also an umbrella term used to refer to any of the three wikis running on the separate networks at different classification levels: the Joint Worldwide Intelligence Communication System (JWICS; Intellipedia-TS), SIPRNet (Intellipedia-S), and DNI-U (Intellipedia-U). Individuals with appropriate clearances and access to the classified networks may be granted access to any of the three wikis by the U.S. intelligence community or other national-security related organizations, including the combatant commands and certain federal departments.

Intellipedia was developed using a free and open-source wiki software named MediaWiki, which is most notably used for Wikipedia. According to the MediaWiki homepage, "MediaWiki is written in the PHP programming language and stores all text content into a database. The software is scalable and optimized to efficiently handle large projects, which can have terabytes of content and hundreds of thousands of views per second."[28] Therefore, there are minimal barriers to developing a GHE Intellipedia using MediaWiki.

For setting up a GHE Intellipedia, we investigated the infrastructure requirements for a secure network, such as Intelink, and an installation of secure wikis using MediaWiki, corresponding to the requirements in the DCR Action 7. However, multiple interactions with GHE practitioners and stakeholders revealed the additional requirement to understand the demand signal for such a collaborative site, particularly because many practitioners at various GCCs had already used the intelligence community's Intellipedia for different purposes. In the next section, we describe the analysis of the responses of GHE practitioners and stakeholders.

Intellipedia

On Intellipedia, users are allowed to create pages arranged by topic that are moderated by SMEs. Users and organizations are also allowed to create homepages, which act as initial points of reference. Similar to other wiki instantiations, this results in broad-ranging subject matter without a particular goal for the knowledge. This style of collaboration has been referred to as crowdsourcing.[29] Intellipedia is only one system made available by Intelink to users on SIPRNet. Intelink also supports several other collaboration tools, which are available on Intelink-U, Intelink-S, or Top Secret/Sensitive Compartmentalized Information (TS/SCI). These include the following:

- **IntelShare.** This instantiation of Microsoft SharePoint is one of the most popular among users. Primarily used by already defined teams, IntelShare assists with collaboration and version control when working on documents, briefings, spreadsheets, etc.
- **Search.** Analogous to Google on classified networks, Intelink Search has more than 180 unique URLs indexed, including products from the other collaborative tools, and allows users to corroborate information or research information gaps.

---

[28] MediaWiki, homepage, undated.

[29] Treverton, 2016.

- **Gallery and iVideo.** Repositories for photos or videos that could facilitate collaboration.
- **Blog.** Intelink Blogs is also one of most used tools on Intelink. Each blog is managed by an organization that is responsible for the content posted on the blog. Blogs have similar functionality to Intellipedia pages when the blogs are open to the public (provided necessary clearances) and reachable via a search functionality.
- **Email.** Email functionality made available to users at different classification levels.
- **Instant Messaging.** Instant Messaging functionality is available to users at different classification levels.
- **IntelDocs.** IntelDocs is a capability for users to share files and documents.
- **eChirp.** eChirp is the interagency microblogging tool similar to Twitter.[30]

Figure 3.3 (adapted from Treverton, 2016), provides a comparison of these Intelink intelligence community collaborative tools with those offered by MedCOP (described in the next section). The figure reflects the active tools available on Intelink described above.

MedCOP

In the prior section, we described the MedCOP platform in greater detail. In this section, we will focus on two applications on the AIDE operating system that support MedCOP: AIDE Drive and CEREBRO. The broad overview of MedCOP capabilities is provided in the previous section on mission data systems.

FIGURE 3.3
Intelink and MedCOP Collaborative Tool Comparison

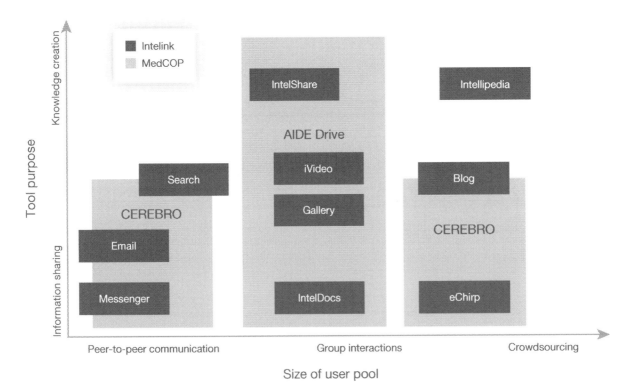

SOURCE: Adapted from Treverton, 2016, p. 14.

---

[30] Treverton, 2016, p. 14

AIDE Drive is a file management system in the AIDE operating system. Files on AIDE Drive can be shared across organizations to the individual level. Files can also be tagged geospatially. Figure 3.3 shows that AIDE Drive mimics the capability of IntelDocs, Gallery, and iVideo, but it has significant overlap with IntelShare as well. CEREBRO is a social media application on the AIDE operating system that provides several capabilities: (1) a social media environment that is similar in capability to Intelink Blog or eChirp and (2) posting and chat capabilities similar to Intelink Email and Messenger. CEREBRO works in sync with the mission command tool and COP, allowing for real-time updates with GeoTag communications.[31]

We should note that an identical Intellipedia capability is not present on the AIDE operating system. However, there are many qualities in Intellipedia and Blog that overlap with Intellipedia. The primary difference between the two is ownership. Wiki-like pages are openly maintained by the broad community who have access to the wiki, and Blogs are maintained by an individual or organization. As a result, the content on Blogs is susceptible to editorial bias, whereas wiki-like content is intended for the internal use of a community (in this case, the global GHE community), resulting in more-objective and encyclopedic content. It is possible to tailor Blogs to mimic wiki content, but this would require some level of oversight or enforcement.

Using MedCOP as a crowdsourcing collaboration platform is not without challenges. Similar to Intelink Blog or Intellipedia, the quality of CEREBRO blog pages is dependent on the level of effort the GHE community is willing to dedicate. This would require the blog pages to be actively maintained and would require the GHE community to "buy into" the MedCOP platform, such that there is a thriving and active user base. Another challenge with using MedCOP is that there are no GHE data currently on the platform. GHE data must be exported from an activity management system, such as Socium, CFR, or OHASIS. As mentioned in previous sections, the MedCOP development team is working with GHE stakeholders to automate the data transfer process. If the integration of GHE data is made available, MedCOP could provide the ability for a COP, data analysis or visualization and analytics, and collaborative tools on a single operating system.

Joint Lessons Learned Information System

JLLIS is "the DoD system of record and enterprise solution developed to support the Chairman of the Joint Chief of Staff's Joint Lessons Learned Process (JLLP). JLLIS facilitates the collection, tracking, management, sharing, collaborative resolution and dissemination of lessons learned to improve the development/readiness of the Joint Force."[32] JLLIS is directly linked to the Defense Readiness Reporting System and is available on NIPR, SIPR, and JWICS. JLLIS provides "automated workflow processes to elevate observations from operations, exercises, training, experiments, and real-world events and facilitates the discovery, validation, issue resolution, evaluation, and dissemination of critical lessons."[33] In total, JLLIS has approximately 6,600 users and 480,000 lessons learned observations.[34]

Users of JLLIS are categorized as general users, lesson managers, and administrators. Administrators are the primary JLLIS point of contact and have the authority to start organization and assign the initial lesson managers. Lessons managers then serve as organizational-level SMEs on the JLLP and manage the organizational-level lessons learned program. The structure of observation data entered and the required accompanying documents entered into JLLIS are not mandated by administrators but instead by the organi-

---

[31] Novetta, 2021.

[32] Chairman of the Joint Chiefs of Staff Manual 3150.25B, *Joint Lessons Learned Program*, Joint Chiefs of Staff, October 2018, p. C-1.

[33] Gwendolyn R. DeFilippi, Stephen Francis Nowak, and Bradford Harlow Baylor, "The Importance of Lessons Learned in Joint Force Development," *Joint Force Quarterly*, No. 89, April 2018, p. 87.

[34] Discussion with JLLIS SME, March 2021.

zation and organization lesson managers. A search of GHE-related observations within JLLIS reveals underutilization by the GHE community, with approximately 160 lessons learned observations. Historically, the GHE-related lesson learned observations are reported to their respective combatant command or combat support agencies organization, making them non-uniform and less accessible to the wider GHE community. Because of variance in how observations are reported across organizations, there is a lack of standardization for the GHE community, which operates across various combatant commands.[35]

JLLIS is in the process of updating the system to JLLIS Next. OSD and the Joint Staff have described improvements to the analytics capabilities, integrating AI and improvements to the cyber infrastructure.[36]

JLLP Community of Practice

The JLLP Community of Practice is a tool within JLLIS that fosters collaboration and interoperability across DoD organizations. The Community of Practice provides a space to post announcements, share and organize data, and contribute to discussion boards. Although a Community of Practice is unable to enforce how observations are entered into JLLIS, the ability to disseminate information that has a common interest and/or that demonstrates or employs similar core competencies may be valuable for GHE, further contributing "information that improves joint capabilities and readiness."[37]

Analysis of Business Value and Technical Quality of Current GHE Platforms

Figure 3.4 uses the assessment model described in Chapter 1 to plot the output of the two scorecards in the decision matrix provided in Tables 2.1 and 3.2. The GHE platforms whose consolidated business value and technical quality fall into the "High Business Value, High Technical Quality" quadrant are Socium and MedCOP.[38] As described in Table 1.2, such systems are candidates for continuous enhancements and should be "actively evolved."[39] In Table 4.1, we provide a more detailed comparison between Socium and MedCOP as the recommended platforms for GHE activities. We also provide recommendations for ensuring that GHE-specific requirements are met by these platforms in current and future enhancements.

---

[35] Discussion with JLLIS SME, March 2021.

[36] Discussion with JLLIS SME, March 2021.

[37] Chairman of the Joint Chiefs of Staff Instruction 3150.25H, 2021, p. A-1.

[38] As noted earlier, the scores for MedCOP were based on the stakeholder inputs on features that were planned to be added to MedCOP and the technical value of the current features and infrastructure of MedCOP that could be customized for the GHE community requirements.

[39] Seacord, Plakosh, and Lewis, 2003, p. 30

FIGURE 3.4

Existing Platforms: Business Value, Technical Quality Decision Matrix

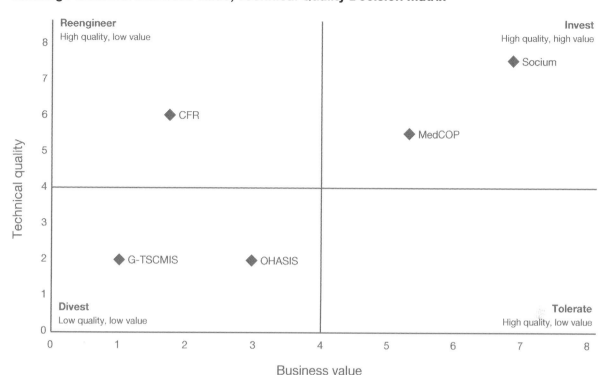

Feasibility of Joint GHE Intellipedia

Despite a robust set of tools available on Intelink, including Intellipedia, the network's user pool outside of the intelligence community is limited. Even within the intelligence community, the information shared on Intellipedia is sparse and often incomplete.[40] Treverton, 2016, among other authors, attributes this to the culture of U.S. intelligence organizations, stating that "'sharing' often is reduced to the minimum necessary: analysts may use search tools to locate fellow experts but then take the communication offline, so that both experts can protect their personal and organizational equities."[41] The sharing of data and information on collaborative platforms requires a degree of trust and openness that conflicts with a closed and controlled classified environment.[42] As mentioned earlier, GHE practitioners at various GCCs have used the intelligence community's Intellipedia to create sites and homepages for specific purposes. However, these sites are no longer maintained or enhanced. There is very little incentive or demand for using a wiki-based information site in the GHE community. Getting a GHE user base to actively maintain and support Intellipedia pages would not be sustainable in the long term.

Additionally, to meet other requirements, GHE users would have to use several tools available on Intelink, such as IntelShare for document sharing. Both the GHE practitioner inputs and the demand signal for these tools indicate that these tools are not easy to access and use. GHE practitioners also prefer a single platform that provides an integrated set of tools. MedCOP provides this integration. Finally, in addition to document sharing (playbooks, doctrine, policies), GHE stakeholders have expressed an interest in an integrated view

---

[40] Discussion with RAND intelligence community experts, multiple dates.

[41] Treverton, 2016, p. 7.

[42] Treverton, 2016.

of the lessons learned from previous GHE activities. MedCOP's integration with a lessons learned platform, such as JLLIS, would be a viable solution for this requirement, particularly for historical engagement data.

CHAPTER 4

Findings and Recommendations

Findings

Our analysis revealed barriers in conducting GHE activities effectively and efficiently and in showcasing the value of GHE in supporting U.S. national security objectives to DoD and the U.S. Congress. Our findings reveal that key stakeholder requirements and concerns are not addressed by the current IT platforms used by the GHE community across GCCs, as discussed in Chapters 2 and 3. Current platforms lack the support for a standardized process of capturing and tracking, accessing, and monitoring information on global health engagements and activities related to all funding streams and exercises. Information is captured in disparate stovepiped systems and is not standardized, verifiable, or complete. Additionally, lack of visibility into GHE information across GCCs is hindering the long-term GHE planning, data analytics, and capability development processes. For a GHE Intellipedia, the consensus of all GHE stakeholders has been that although a collaborative platform that provides shared resources, intelligence, and tools for partnerships or sharing across GCCs is required, an Intellipedia-like site might not be the answer. GHE stakeholders preferred to have support for collaboration within the platforms used for GHE activities. We summarize our findings in this section, followed by our recommendations.

Findings for Technology Platform Assessment (Action 9)

Current technology platforms do not support all GHE practitioners' requirements for capturing and tracking all activities. The GHE community of practitioners uses multiple technology platforms to capture and track GHE activities. Information on various activities and funding streams is captured in disparate stovepiped systems (e.g., CFR, G-TSCMIS, and the Cloud-Based Traditional Combatant Command Activities [TCA] Information Management System [CTIMS]; described in Appendix D). This does not serve the need for a flexible platform to capture "all medical things," automate reporting requirements, and improve AM&E capabilities.

GHE missions and activities vary based on funding sources and the region of operation, since GHE practitioners must use several funding streams according to the needs and parameters of the health engagement with the partner. Some of the examples of funding used by GHE include funding related to security cooperation programs (Title 10, Title 22), humanitarian assistance (OHDACA), short-term activities, GHE activities within a military-to-military exercise, and component- and partner-funded projects. Hence, with different funding streams, practitioners at various GCCs and component commands have to capture and track funding requests and activities in different systems and sometimes even in spreadsheets, documents, and local or SharePoint locations, resulting in dispersed tracking of and information on global health engagements. Table D.1 lists the technology platforms used by GHE practitioners.

GHE planners' and practitioners' requirements for technology platforms can be categorized into the ability to (1) capture and track activities in a single system or multiple systems that integrate data across multiple sources, (2) access applicable policies and doctrines related to funding authority and host-nation capabilities and (3) upgrade the platform based on end-user inputs.

Current platforms are not user-friendly, are not consistently maintained, and lack data standardization. GHE practitioners have found security cooperation (GHE) platforms, particularly those mandated as the authoritative data platforms for security cooperation (for example, G-TSCMIS), to be not user-friendly. Even for the first release of the Socium platform, the general view can be summarized as follows: The platform is not easy to use, does not solve the issue of integrating all data systems or funding authorities into one platform, and does not support many of the various funding authority life cycles or process workflows, such as the 10 U.S.C. § 312 funding authority.[1] In addition, the mandates on data entry are not easy to enforce. This leads to missing data. There is, however, a recognition in the community of a need for a change in culture and more-enforceable mandates (such as repercussions for noncompliance).

A comprehensive GHE platform also needs to include the following incentives: (1) support for all GHE related funding authorities, (2) a plan for integration with more "data systems," both homegrown application platforms and GHE activity data captured outside application platforms, (3) capabilities to view all the activities in the GCC AOR and across all GCCs, and (4) alignment of features and process workflows with funding and outcomes.

GHE practitioners have limited access to historical data and information on current GHE engagements and limited visibility into all GHE activities within one and across all AORs. Current GHE activities are stovepiped with little context or insight into the planned or ongoing GHE engagements of other service component commands or of NGOs and non-DoD agencies within the AOR and across all AORs. Additionally, GHE practitioners do not have access to much of the historical data on previous global health engagements.

GHE planners and practitioners expressed the need for the following:

- access to historical information on previous funding, missions, and activities, AARs, and GHE proposals that have been approved; this kind of information would provide useful templates when drafting a proposal or funding requests (classification levels considered)—for example, for OHDACA or Title 10 funding authorities
- insight into current activities within a GCC AOR and across all GCCs for measuring effectiveness across GCCs
- insight into historical, approved, and ongoing activities of NGOs and other agencies within the GCC AOR to avoid overlaps, redundancy, or gaps while facilitating stepwise, sequential capability-building in partner nations.

> "The issue is making sure we are capturing all the medical things that are going on, which can be difficult when there are so many players."
> SOURCE: GHE SME discussion, January 7, 2021.

The GHE community seeks an integrated (and, ideally, a single) platform that would help with data access and visibility across GCCs, interoperability, sharing lessons learned, and cost analysis. Although many GHE stakeholders recognized the complexity of capturing global health engagements related to various funding authorities, sources, and activities embedded within component command exercises, a single system that captures all GHE activities is considered ideal for supporting the various GHE functions of plan-

---

[1] Stakeholder discussions conducted in 2020 and 2021. Socium has since added support for the generic workflow to make data entry easier, among other features.

ning, tracking, assessing, and reporting GHE activities. Additionally, such a system would provide a single source of information for the leadership and for showcasing the value of GHE.

Mandates and policies must support GHE practitioners and better data capturing practices. The biggest challenge for consistent data entry, verification, and assessment and analysis on GHE activities may be enforcing mandatory use of any "authoritative" security cooperation or GHE platform. One of the drawbacks of G-TSCMIS was that a significant amount of data were missing, even with a mandatory requirement for entering all data related to security cooperation or global health engagements. There also was a generic lack of understanding of data entities and for the data required for NIPR and SIPR network instances of G-TSCMIS. This was due to a lack of data standards or data entry guidelines. The system did not provide automatic verification. Additionally, most data are from component programs or military-to-military engagements and therefore are captured in GCC-funded homegrown systems. Although some homegrown systems, such as EUCOM's CFR platform, have a robust life-cycle management support, dedicated funding, and dedicated maintenance and enhancement teams, not all GHE practitioners at various GCCs have access to comparable systems. Enforcement of mandates must be accompanied by policies, resources, ease of use, and support for multiple funding streams.

Data analytics capabilities are needed for showcasing the value of GHE to combatant commanders, the Joint Chiefs of Staff, DoD civilian leadership and the U.S. Congress. GHE decisionmakers, planners, and practitioners see enormous value in integrating the data for GHE missions and activities and supporting advanced analytics capabilities. The immediate value of an analytics platform are seen as (1) providing a COP of global health engagements to determine measures of performance, measures of effectiveness, and return on investment (2) highlighting the importance of including GHE in TCPs and global campaign plans, (3) showcasing the relevance of GHE to GCCs and the Joint Force, including the benefit of improving the readiness of U.S. forces and partner forces and as an effective tool for building and sustaining partnerships, (4) highlighting the engagements that require longer duration or continuous funding, and (5) providing strategic assessment and planning, gap analysis, and information-sharing with other relevant stakeholders, such as the U.S. Agency for International Development, the President's Emergency Plan for AIDS Relief (PEPFAR), the Defense Attaché officers, and GCCs to identify gaps and tailor engagements for a partner or host country.

> "A lot of people just see what we're doing as a bunch of do-gooder stuff."
> SOURCE: GHE SME discussion, January 26, 2021.

Findings for Feasibility of Implementing a Joint GHE Intellipedia (Action 7)

The GHE community sees little value in a separate GHE Intellipedia site because of issues with maintenance and ease of use, despite CAC access. GHE practitioners and stakeholders see value in a collaborative platform that is easy to access and navigate and that is consistently managed, with proper transfer of knowledge between responsible entities. The community would benefit from a platform that supports collaborative tools, such as discussion forums, bulletin boards, document storage for training material (colors of money, GHE and security cooperation objectives, etc.), country information, handbooks, and other virtual interactive tools available across GCCs. Such a platform would be useful for training and educating teams, sharing intelligence, and providing integrated views to the Joint Staff.

Intellipedia was initially considered a "go-to" option for GHE because it is CAC-enabled and was deemed to provide visibility to all GCCs. However, only two or three GHE teams across GCCs have been able to use it with some success, depending on the leadership of the teams at that time. CAC access and early enthusiasm toward Intellipedia were seen as the reasons for the DCR action for the feasibility assessment.

Information shared on previous GCC Intellipedia pages was not intelligence and has been of little use beyond the GCC. Many of the GHE pages developed on the intelligence community's Intellipedia were only landing pages with information on points of contact and were primarily used for advertising events. Many GHE stakeholders viewed the information shared on blogs and pages as information that needed "sifting through" and that provided very little intelligence.

> "If you say . . . you need to go to Poland and if they go to the website and it's just . . . war stories, etc., then it's not efficient. I like the idea of a community of sharing information. [However,] that really wouldn't be utilized."
> SOURCE: GHE SME discussion, January 19, 2021.

GHE practitioners prefer to use an integrated platform that also supports collaborative tools. Because the primary funding and engagement data are captured in dedicated platforms, many GHE practitioners and stakeholders prefer to use a single platform or an integrated set of platforms that also provides collaborative tools. As people rotate between GCCs and component commands, depending on authorities and colors of money, the funding and authorities and means to gather that information would be as important as the intelligence shared about a country and the engagements in a country. For example, DoD routinely goes into an area transiently; therefore, information kept on a database on historical engagements in the area or country would be critical, along with what is shared in a collaborative environment. GCCs could leverage the state partners in these areas, such as the National Guard State Partner Program, that do not change or move every two to three years to gather and share information about the area by providing them the funding, authorities, and means. This could include information on a potential or existing partner country to plan allied and partner cooperation.[2] For example, historical knowledge of the colonial history of Cote D'Ivoire would help in planning the involvement of allies, such as France, during an engagement. GHE practitioners see the value in having these multiple layers of information accessible through an integrated platform instead of a separate GHE Intellipedia site.

Recommendations

From our analysis of GHE stakeholder requirements and the technical quality of platforms (Chapters 2 and 3), we find that there are several possible actions OASD(HA) and the GCCs should take to support GHE practitioners and activities and to increase the effectiveness and efficiency of GHE worldwide.

Recommendations for a GHE Integrated Platform (Action 9)

Recommendation 1: OASD(HA) should facilitate the creation of a GHE Integrated Product Team (IPT) to provide GHE-specific platform requirements and acceptance criteria to system developers. The GHE community, including GHE practitioners, planners, and other relevant stakeholders to the primary platform(s) used by the GHE community (as noted in the following recommendation), should be actively engaged with system developers as they develop GHE-specific enhancements. The GHE community in such IPTs would ensure that the platform has support for relevant process workflows and life-cycle management,

---

[2]   Discussion with GHE SME, January 19, 2021.

along with user-friendly interfaces and templates. The GHE community should define the acceptance criteria for relevant process workflows and should specify data integration (DoD and external data sets) and analytics requirements for the identified platform. If Socium is the identified platform, a data integration with MedCOP for analytics support would allow GHE planners and practitioners to leverage existing MedCOP integration with external data sets for a complete COP.

Recommendation 2: The GHE community should leverage existing platforms, with the IPT directing future enhancements, maintenance, and usability. We used our analysis in Chapters 2 and 3 to determine the following pathways for future technology solutions for GHE:

- current platform(s) with enhancements
- a cloud-based integration solution catering to GHE requirements
- de novo platform acquisition.

In our technology assessment of the primary platforms used by the GHE community of practice, we looked at platforms capturing activities related to Title 10 and Title 22 funding sources and those funded by military-to-military and other GCC and component command funding sources. Figure 3.4 illustrates that two current platforms are positioned to support GHE requirements in the future: Socium and MedCOP. Detailed individual assessment of Socium and MedCOP is provided in Chapter 3. Table 4.1 shows a comparison of the two platforms with regard to their current and planned future support for GHE requirements. The GHE community should provide input for enhancements and leverage both these platforms to provide an integrated set of capabilities supported by each of them.

Recommendation 3: The GHE technology platform should provide different process workflows to support different funding and activity needs. GHE planners and our extended research team are investigating the possibility of restructuring the funding of GHE activities to bring all GHE activities under a single funding umbrella.[3] Subject to approval and implementation, this change in GHE funding presents a different set of requirements. Table 4.1 provides a comparison of system features and requirements support in Socium and MedCOP. Depending on the funding structure, either Socium or MedCOP would be better positioned to meet the requirements.

To provide integrated support for GHE activities using the current multiple funding sources, Socium's activity life-cycle workflow design (currently implemented for 10 U.S.C. § 333 and 10 U.S.C. § 345) provides better structural support to implement more workflows for other funding sources. Socium also provides a safety net or stop-gap solution for tracking activities that are not fully implemented in the platform (generic workflow). Socium, however, would still require a data integration with MedCOP for data analytics support that would include external data sets.

To track activities under a new GHE funding umbrella, MedCOP would be better positioned to design and implement a new activity life-cycle management system to track GHE activities. MedCOP currently only supports COP and the analytics requirements of the medical community. It does not have any support for GHE activity life-cycle management. However, MedCOP offers GHE stakeholders an opportunity to define and orchestrate the new system requirements to cater to GHE-specific needs.

Recommendation 4: The platform should support a future GHE funding structure with integrated, accessible, and discoverable historical data on the planning and funding of activities, as well as AARs across all GCCs. In the short term, the GCCs would use many of the current in-house platforms until Socium or MedCOP (Recommendation 2) would have the functional support for all the funding authorities and/or needs of the GHE community. Some in-house platforms may exist even with complete support within

---

[3] The findings and recommendations related to this research (based on actions in the DCR) are in Grill et al., 2023.

TABLE 4.1

Socium and MedCOP Support for GHE Requirements

GHE Platform Needs	Socium	MedCOP
Ease of access to the platform for GHE practitioners across AORs and DoD	Cloud-based (DSCA Cloud) integrated platform available on NIPRNet and SIPRNet (in progress)	Cloud-based (DHA Cloud) Integrated Platform available on NIPRNet and SIPRNet (in progress)
Integration of historical GHE-related activity data	Socium already has a road map of data integration with many systems used for GHE or security cooperation activities, including OHASIS.	MedCOP would be able to support GHE data integration with Socium, OHASIS, and other homegrown systems.
Support all life-cycle activities related to GHE (various funding streams)	Socium supports activity life cycles for 10 U.S.C. § 333 and 10 U.S.C. § 345 authorities. These can be expanded. Socium supports a generic activity management life cycle for other funding sources that do not have support in Socium as of today.	MedCOP would be able to support life-cycle management on the AIDE system. Because MedCOP has no current GHE or security cooperation activity management support, the design of a new GHE life-cycle management interface would allow for direct engagement of GHE stakeholders (IPT) and would follow the least path of resistance. A comprehensive design and implementation plan would be required for creating and tracking the activity life cycle.
Support data analytics capabilities for COP, return on investment, and other assessments of DoD-wide GHE activities	Socium only supports GIS-based analytics. There are no plans to integrate medical data outside GHE activities. Hence, Socium would need an integration with MedCOP for advanced analytics support.	MedCOP provides COP and analytics capabilities with integration of real-time medical data from various programs. It would need integration with Socium and GHE data.
Long-term viability by a Program of Record designation	Program of Record	Not a Program of Record, currently
Continuous support for enhancements and integration	1.5 years in production with Agile continuous integration, continuous deployment (CI/CD) implementation	In production since 2020. Currently has support for non-GHE medical data analysis. Follows Agile CI/CD. Currently has active involvement and interest of GHE stakeholders for future enhancement.
Design maturity	Workflows are designed to map life-cycle management	MedCOP currently does not support GHE workflows. However, at the time of this writing, GHE stakeholders and MedCOP were in discussions about the requirements.
GHE activities using multiple funding sources	Activity life-cycle workflow support for various authorities. Structurally better positioned to reuse design and support activities related to other funding sources.	Would need to design and integrate multiple life-cycle management requirements.
GHE single funding source (if U.S. Congress and OSD approve and implement a single funding source for GHE in the future)	Would require a complex design change to identify or separate activities related to GHE-specific funding	Better positioned to design and implement a life-cycle management to support GHE-specific funding and related mandates
Current GHE IPT or advisors	Informal advisory panel from CGHE, INDOPACOM, and U.S. Navy Medical Services Corps	Very early stages of discussions with GHE stakeholders about creating a formal IPT
Capability for stakeholder engagement in requirements and acceptance criteria for platform	Ongoing for the larger security cooperation organization	Still in development, very early stages
Risk	Workflows are already designed to map life-cycle management. Low risk.	No support for workflows as of today; extent of support on AIDE platform unknown. Higher risk.

NOTE: Information on MedCOP is based on our last engagement with the MedCOP team in November 2021.

a global platform for all types of engagements because of the ease of maintenance and enhancements for a specific GCC-funded platform. As mentioned earlier, Socium's and MedCOP's technology infrastructure and agile development methodology would support the planning and implementation of additional "workflows." Socium already has a road map for the support of multiple workflows, as discussed in Chapter 3, and offers a "generic" workflow to accommodate all other funding authorities that the platform currently does not support.

If GHE activities continue to use the current multiple funding sources, Socium should prioritize and implement separate workflows to support military-to-military 10 U.S.C. § 312 and other funding authorities and their life cycles. This would support those GCCs that do not have a robust in-house system.

Socium or MedCOP should provide mechanisms for data ingestion from such platforms as CFR, OHASIS, and other GHE ad hoc data sources. This would give GHE practitioners access to all historical and current GHE data on various types of engagements.

For Socium (Recommendation 2), the "generic" workflow should be an exception and not a norm: It should be considered only as an interim solution for most of the funding and life cycle needs.

For MedCOP (Recommendation 2), the system should implement a prototype for GHE stakeholders and practitioners, based on the requirements and acceptance criteria provided by the GHE IPT, to allow end-user usability, scalability, and reliability assessments of a new life-cycle management platform on the AIDE operating system.

Recommendation 5: The platform should provide continuous data integration with AOR-specific homegrown systems used by the GHE community and should import data captured in siloed on-premises systems. As mentioned in the previous recommendation, some in-house (or homegrown) platforms within the GCCs may exist even with complete support for all types of engagements in a global platform because of ease of maintenance and enhancements for a specific GCC-funded platform. Hence, Socium or MedCOP should provide continuous data integration mechanisms for such systems as CFR, OHASIS, CTIMS, and other GHE ad hoc data sources to ensure visibility of all captured data and data consistency across GCCs. Continuous data integration would also support advanced analytical capabilities and a COP of all GHE activities.

Recommendation 6: The platform should include data entry compliance and verification to ensure the completeness of ongoing and after-action updates of GHE activities. The GHE IPT should specify the required data compliance mandates and policies for the completeness of GHE activity information. The GHE technology platform should include these mandates and policies within the activity workflow interfaces as mandatory data entry checks. This will address the issue of missing data and lack of data entry checks, as seen in G-TSCMIS. Additionally, to ensure that all required activity data are captured, the GHE IPT should consider the following verification requirements for the identified platform:

- The workflow should be directly tied to funding and life-cycle management, including approvals, tracking, and AAR updates for completeness. In other words, funding would be approved only when the requisite data are tracked, entered, and verified throughout the life cycle of an engagement.
- Appropriate training on platform use and compliance with system needs should be mandated.

Recommendation 7: The GHE IPT should continuously monitor and communicate data and verification policies with the platform program management. The GHE IPT should be the authoritative source of all data-capturing and data verification policies to facilitate current and future planned global health engagements, as well as for all GHE platform requirements, enhancements, and acceptance criteria.

Recommendation 8: GHE platform(s) should provide advanced data analytics capabilities that leverage integrated GHE data to enable reporting, forecasting, planning, and decisionmaking for GHE leadership. Socium and MedCOP both provide GIS-based analytic support. For more-comprehensive analytics and decisionmaking support, including data engineering and AI-based capabilities, an integrated effort supporting data flows to leverage Socium's data integration with other platforms and MedCOP's analytical tools is recommended.

Recommendations from the Study on Implementing a Joint GHE Intellipedia (Action 7)

Recommendation 9: Because there is no demand signal for a separate GHE Intellipedia-like site, the GHE community should consider other integrated platform alternatives to facilitate collaboration and knowledge- and intelligence-sharing. GHE stakeholders and practitioners do not see any value in the investment in and maintenance of a new GHE Intellipedia site. Additionally, the community prefers a single platform that supports GHE activities and a set of collaborative tools and document repositories. This would allow easy maintenance of the platform and tools. This would also ensure that data shared within these collaborative tools would not be obsolete and would be easily available to multiple practitioners with the right authentication and authorization credentials. As discussed in Chapter 3, the GHE community should consider the comparable tools provided by MedCOP for collaboration in an integrated platform.

Recommendation 10: The GHE community should explore the integration of data from platforms capturing lessons learned, AARs, and information on other joint events. To support the need for document and resource accessibility in an Intellipedia-like site, the GHE community should explore the integration of lessons learned and AAR data from such platforms as JLLIS, as well as information on joint and allied partnership events from other systems used by the GHE community.

Conclusion

There is an emphasis on using COTS products where possible because using such products is considered a cost-effective way of acquiring a capability. Reducing costs and downsizing management and technical personnel makes COTS products preferable over the maintenance and enhancement of in-house products. Although this has been true for many DoD systems for nearly two decades, COTS products do not provide immediate advantages for both cost and capability. This is because DoD platforms require special feature support that does not come out of the box with many commercial systems: for example, support for policies and regulations specific to the organization within DoD.[4] GHE activity workflows, workflows of the engagements of the greater security cooperation organization, and workflows embedded within component command exercises all require new designs or tailoring product functionality. Regardless of the cost and effort involved in implementing a new COTS product for a specific need, it is imperative to analyze the current systems for their business value and technical quality to establish the benefits or drawbacks of maintaining and enhancing an existing system. In this report, we used a model to assess platforms used by the GHE community to establish the platforms that provide high business value and high technical quality. These platforms are candidates for enhancements to support future GHE requirements instead of customizing a new COTS platform exclusively for GHE activities.

In this report, we also looked into the need and feasibility of a GHE Intellipedia for intelligence- and knowledge-sharing and collaboration. With many platforms providing app-based collaborative tools, such as MedCOP, the need and demand for a wiki-based Intellipedia site is minimal for the GHE community. As the GHE community looks for an integrated platform that will support planning, funding, recording, and track-

---

[4]   Carol Sledge and David Carney, "Case Study: Evaluating COTS Products for DoD Information Systems," Software Engineering Institute, Carnegie Mellon University, June 1998.

ing GHE activities, GHE stakeholders should include the requirement for collaborative tools and document repositories to the integrated platform requirements. As our analysis recommends, an integrated platform of Socium and MedCOP with data exchange with other significant GHE platforms would support all the requirement of the GHE practitioners, planners, and DoD leadership.

We recommend two GHE end-user case studies as a follow-up to this study at different GCCs to capture the requirements and concerns of the end users of these platforms. This would help identify the processes needed for a continuous feedback loop and to establish a stakeholder community that interacts with the GHE IPT to address the end-user needs.

With this study, we could not examine the data analytics needs to recommend specific related capabilities. Further studies on the use cases for advanced analytics would be beneficial to understand data standardization, data engineering, and analytics requirements and benefits for the GHE leadership.

Finally, one of the requirements that was categorized as "nice-to-have" for this study was support for automatic incorporation of data captured in handheld devices on the field into an integrated GHE platform. We could not assess the current capabilities and potential for future enhancements to support this requirement because of platform management having other features with higher priorities in the pipeline. A future study in this area would be useful to enhance the support for end users of GHE platforms.

Discussion Protocols

This appendix documents the protocols developed for conducting semistructured discussions for this research. As described in Chapter 2, we developed two protocols. The first is for GHE stakeholders and practitioners to garner their inputs related to the DCR actions researched for this project. This protocol sought to obtain information on the current platforms, bottlenecks and issues, and future requirements from GHE practitioners based on the research questions identified (Chapter 1). The second protocol is for program managers and program leads for the various IT platforms used by the GHE community, as well those in production. For questions related to Intellipedia and Intelink, we created another version of the protocol for program managers. We then derived platform requirements using a coding and content analysis approach, as described in Chapter 2.

Subject-Matter Expert and Stakeholder Discussion Protocol

RAND NDRI Study: GLOBAL HEALTH ENGAGEMENT—IMPROVING SUPPORT TO COMBATANT COMMANDS
Draft Discussion Protocol
1. INTRODUCTION AND VERBAL CONSENT

Thank you for taking the time to speak with us today. We're from the RAND Corporation, a nonprofit, nonpartisan institution that conducts research on behalf of the U.S. government, private institutions, and foreign governments. With your permission, I'll begin by introducing the members of the RAND study team, providing you with some background on our research study, and giving you an opportunity to ask any preliminary questions before we start our discussion. My name is_____. I will lead the discussion today. My colleagues, _____, will assist me in conducting the discussion. _____will be taking notes but will only be sharing our notes with members of our team. The principal investigators for the study are Dr. Trupti Brahmbhatt and Dr. Jennifer Moroney.

The study came about as a result of the 2018 GHE Capability Based Assessment (CBA) to facilitate efficient conduct of GHE activities and is sponsored by the Office of the Assistant Secretary of Defense for Health Affairs (OASD[HA]). OASD(HA) asked RAND to assess Global Health Engagement (GHE) education and training, technology platforms, and funding mechanisms to help DoD synchronize GHE training and education and enable long-term GHE capability development for the Combatant Commands (CCMDs). Our project monitor in the Health Affairs office is Dr. Chris Daniel, the senior advisor for Global Health Engagement.

We selected you in consultation with our sponsor because of your experience in the global health engagement field. Although we believe your insights will be quite valuable, you are of course free to decline to participate in the discussion, decline to answer any question, and to provide the level of detail you feel is appropriate.

You should also know that while we will be taking notes during the discussion, your responses will remain anonymous. We will be presenting themes and variation in responses across discussions in our study report for OASD(HA). We may include some direct quotes but will not be attributing them to anyone by name or position in a way that would directly identify you.

Do you have any questions at this time? Would you like to continue with the discussion?

2. BACKGROUND QUESTIONS

We would like to begin by asking some questions about your GHE-related experience.

1. Would you please indicate the major DoD (or other USG or non-USG) organization you currently belong to (e.g., OSD, Joint Staff, Geographic Combatant Command, Service headquarters)?
2. Would you please describe your current position as well as any GHE-related responsibilities or interests related to this position?
3. How many years of GHE-related experience do you have? Would you briefly describe this experience?
4. Have you received any GHE-related training and education? If so, who was the provider? In what ways has this training and education helped you in carrying out subsequent GHE responsibilities? In what ways has it been insufficient? Examples would be helpful.

3. GENERAL QUESTIONS

Next, we would like to ask you some general questions about the GHE enterprise.

1. From your perspective, what are DoD's top GHE priorities?
2. How and to what extent do GHE priorities support global and theater objectives?
3. What are the primary types of GHE capabilities that DoD and the CCMDs are seeking to develop over the long term?
4. What challenges, if any, do you see in enabling long-term support of GHE-related CCMD objectives?

4. FUNDING QUESTIONS

We would now like to ask a few questions related to the funding of GHE activities.

1. What types of GHE activities are you currently conducting or overseeing?
2. Who are your primary governmental partners in planning, resourcing, or executing these activities?
3. What are the primary authorities and sources of funding used to support these GHE activities?
4. What challenges, if any, are the CCMDs and GHE providers facing in using current authorities and funding sources? What can't they do based on the authority or funding limitations if anything?
5. If some changes are required, what types of funding mechanisms would more effectively support CCMD objectives?
6. Do you currently track GHE activities and funding? If so, how? Is this system working well for your office? If not, what changes would you suggest, if any?

5. TRAINING AND EDUCATION QUESTIONS

We would now like to ask you some questions related to the training and education of DoD personnel in GHE topics.

1. What specific groups within DoD require some form of GHE training and education?
2. What GHE-related knowledge, skills and abilities does each group need?
   a. Who defines these needs?
   b. Based on whose requirements?

3. Are the aforementioned groups currently receiving GHE-related training and education?

4. Which institutions should be responsible for executing GHE training and education for different groups of DoD personnel?

5. What challenges, if any, exist to offering appropriate GHE-related training and education to different groups of DoD personnel? To what extent can these challenges be overcome? If so, how?

6. QUESTIONS ON INFORMATION SYSTEMS

1. Please tell us about the current information systems that your organization is using.

2. Who are the main users—producers and consumers of information of these systems—within your organization and in the wider GHE enterprise?

3. Would the availability/access to any additional information or data help in enabling more effective GHE planning?

4. What would be helpful during an IT systems upgrade, desired features, or functions? Why are these new upgrades, features, or functions so critical?

5. Do you envision any specific technological upgrades, such as cloud/data centers or analytical tools (including AI), that may increase the collaboration and effectiveness of the GHE community (similar to the ongoing effort with Socium)?

7. QUESTIONS ON JOINT GHE INTELLIPEDIA SITE

GHE is exploring the development of a joint GHE "Intellipedia" site, similar to the one used by the U.S. intelligence agencies.

1. Assuming that an access-controlled site would be available on both NIPR and SIPR, would your organization benefit from the information on such a site (in addition to the IT systems already in place)?

2. How would this type of platform improve the collaboration among the GHE community?

8. CONCLUDING QUESTIONS

As we wrap up, we would now like to ask you:

1. Is there anything else we did not cover that we should consider?

2. Are there any other individuals or organizations you feel we should speak to who have good visibility on these issues and could provide valuable insights for our study? Would you kindly provide their contact information?

3. Is there any documentation you could share with us that you think would be relevant?

Platform and Application Program Management Discussion Protocol

1. What type of information or data is required to enable effective GHE planning?
   a. Is this information or data readily available to you on an existing IT system? If not, how do you access it?
   b. Are these databases managed in house? Could you speak to the upkeep of these databases (or provide a point of contact for who is responsible for the input, administration, and verification of the data; frequency of changes)?

2. With what other organizations do you collaborate with to exchange relevant expertise, innovate, and share lessons learned?
   a. What is the medium you currently use to collaborate?
   b. Are there any requirements this communication medium struggles to satisfy?

    c.   How do you foresee partner nations involvement with GHE IT systems (uploading of source information, communication channels, access to classified/unclassified, etc.)?

3.   How would your organization utilize an Intellipedia-like system?

    a.   What essential requirements need to be fulfilled in order for an Intellipedia-like system to be effective?

    b.   What challenges do you foresee in using and maintaining Intellipedia pages?

4.   What are your thoughts on utilizing a cloud-based services for database systems and data analytic solutions?

    a.   What is the feasibility of migrating existing database systems to a single cloud-based system?

    b.   Are there any data analytic requirements which must be met by a prospective cloud-based system? (Machine learning, big data, etc.)

5.   Are there any other existing technology products and platforms utilized by your organization?

6.   Are there any additional challenges you expect when using any current or future GHE information management system discussed today?

Intellipedia Program and Project Management Discussion Protocol

RAND NDRI Study: GLOBAL HEALTH ENGAGEMENT—IMPROVING SUPPORT TO COMBATANT COMMANDS

Draft Discussion Protocol

1. INTRODUCTION AND VERBAL CONSENT

Thank you for taking the time to speak with us today. We're from the RAND Corporation, a nonprofit, non-partisan institution that conducts research on behalf of the U.S. government, private institutions, and foreign governments. With your permission, I'll begin by introducing the members of the RAND study team, providing you with some background on our research study, and giving you an opportunity to ask any preliminary questions before we start our discussion. My name is_____. I will lead the discussion today. My colleagues, _____, will assist me in conducting the discussion. _____will be taking notes but will only be sharing our notes with members of our team. The principal investigators for the study are Dr. Trupti Brahmbhatt and Dr. Jennifer Moroney.

The study came about as a result of the 2018 Global Health Engagement (GHE) Capability Based Assessment (CBA) to facilitate efficient conduct of GHE activities and is sponsored by the Office of the Assistant Secretary of Defense for Health Affairs (OASD[HA]). OASD(HA) has asked RAND to assess Global Health Engagement (GHE) technology platforms to enable long-term GHE capability development for the Combatant Commands (CCMDs). One of the focus areas of our study would be to assess the requirements and the feasibility of setting up a GHE-wide collaborative data sharing system, similar to Intellipedia. Our project monitor is Dr. Chris Daniel, Health Affairs office, the senior advisor for Global Health Engagement.

We have selected you in consultation with our sponsor because of your experience in the design and/or the development of the Intellipedia system for the U.S. Intelligence Community. Although we believe your insights will be quite valuable, you are of course free to decline to participate in the discussion, decline to answer any question, and to provide the level of detail you feel is appropriate.

You should also know that while we will be taking notes during the discussion, your responses will remain anonymous. We will be presenting themes and variation in responses across discussions in our study report for OASD(HA). We may include some direct quotes but will not be attributing them to anyone by name or position in a way that would directly identify you.

Do you have any questions at this time? Would you like to continue with the discussion?

2. BACKGROUND QUESTIONS
QUESTIONS RELATED TO THE INTELLIPEDIA SITE

GHE is exploring the development of a joint GHE "Intellipedia" like site The GHE site will be an access-controlled site that would be available on NIPRNet and SIPRNet, depending upon the classification of the content being shared.

1. Based on your experience with the development of Intellipedia and use by the Intelligence Community, how would you see this type of platform improving the collaboration among the GHE community? What are the features that could be offered by such a system that would be different from any other data management and data visualization interfaces?
2. Have you experienced/received feedback from the users about the advantages of using a Wikipedia style free form information sharing? Could you share them with us?
3. Are there any significant differences between the activities on the SIPRNet and the unclassified versions, in terms of the number of users, information shared, information audit, attribution and peer-review processes other than the classification itself?
4. Could you tell us about the design and the technology stack used for setting up the Intellipedia system on the Intelink network, both for the unclassified and, if possible, for the classified versions.
5. What challenges do you envision in setting up a similar system for GHE—the network requirements as well as building a Wikipedia-style content sharing site(s).
6. How does Intellipedia balance the "need to know" security requirement with a system built for collaborative, explorative data sharing, and disseminating material?
7. We have seen a relatively rapid adoption of Intellipedia in the intelligence community. Was there initial resistance? How did Intellipedia developers get buy-in from the community at large?
8. Could you speak to the formal training programs implemented and whether the programs effectively convinced potential users?

CONCLUDING QUESTIONS

As we wrap up, we would now like to ask you:

1. Is there anything else we did not cover that we should consider?
2. Are there any other individuals or organizations you feel we should speak to who have good visibility on these issues and could provide valuable insights for our study? Would you kindly provide their contact information?
3. Is there any documentation you could share with us that you think would be relevant?

3. ADDITIONAL INTELLIPEDIA QUESTIONS:

1. How would you describe the distribution of articles and users across the three levels of classification?
   a. In your opinion, is there a reason why top-secret version on SIPR-Net has the most users and content?
      i. Are there limitations in the view of the users to the SECRET or UNCLASS level Intellipedia which make them non-ideal?
   b. Do users at different classification levels interact in a different way depending on the level of classification? (i.e., More open to discussions on methods, analysis, critical feedback, etc.)
2. How does Intellipedia balance the "need to know" security requirement with a system built for collaborative, explorative data sharing, and disseminating material?
3. We have seen a relatively rapid adoption of Intellipedia in the intelligence community. Was there initial resistance? How did Intellipedia developers get buy-in from the community at large?

      a.   Could you speak to the formal training programs implemented and whether the programs effectively convinced potential users?

4.   Are there concerns that individual intelligence agencies (like GHE) creating their own wikis, draining ideas and input from Intellipedia?

      a.   Are there examples of other individual agencies creating their own wiki? Are any still in use or successful that you know of?

5.   Does Intellipedia enforce quality control on articles or moderate discussions?

      a.   Could you elaborate on why this decision was made?

6.   Did Intellipedia consider other forms of communication between users (other than through discussion pages, i.e., direct user message)?

Coding and Content Analysis Framework

Tables B.1 and B.2 provide the frameworks used in our analysis.

TABLE B.1

GHE Community (Stakeholder) Discussion Analysis Framework

Stakeholder Organizations	Contact Name(s)	Assessment: Current Systems and Requirements																
		G-TSCMIS	GIS	JLLIS	OHASIS	CFR	ADVANA	APAN	NCMI	DIA	SOCIUM	Positive Features	Requirements	Bottlenecks	Nice to Haves	Intellipedia	Response
CGHE Liaison: EUCOM and AFRICOM																	
U.S. Army Veterinary Corps																	
DSCA/BPC/ HDM																	
AFRICOM Command Surgeon																	
CENTCOM Command Surgeon																	
BUMED																	
INDOPACOM Command Surgeon																	
SOUTHCOM																	
INDOPACOM GHE Branch Chief																	
Army Medical Corps Services Officer																	
U.S. Air Force International Health Program																	

Table B.1—Continued

Stakeholder Organizations	Contact Name(s)	Assessment: Current Systems and Requirements														
		G-TSCMIS	GIS	JLLIS	OHASIS	CFR	ADVANA	APAN	NCMI	DIA	SOCIUM	Positive Features	Requirements	Bottlenecks	Nice to Haves	Intellipedia Response
CENTCOM																
EUCOM Command Surgeon																
CGHE Director																
PACAF Command Surgeon																
SOCSOUTH																
Joint Staff Surgeon and OASD(HA)																

NOTE: BPC = Building Partner Capacity Directorate; BUMED = Navy Bureau of Medicine and Surgery; HDM = Humanitarian Assistance, Disaster Relief, and Mine Action; PACAF = Pacific Air Forces; SOCSOUTH = Special Operations Command South.

TABLE B.2
System Analysis Framework

	G-TSCMIS	GIS	JLLIS	OHASIS	CFR	ADVANA	APAN	NCMI	DSCA IM&T	SOCIUM
Management Strategy										
Vision										
Management strategy										
Organization procedures										
Technological dependencies										
Technological coverage degree										
System Features										
Process management										
Process procedures										
Process efficiency										
Legality										
Maintenance record										
Technological support quality										
System Analysis										
Portability										
Maturity										
Interoperability										
Adequacy										
Architecture										
Size										
Security										
Data dependencies										

Table B.2—Continued

	G-TSCMIS	GIS	JLLIS	OHASIS	CFR	ADVANA	APAN	NCMI	DSCA IM&T	SOCIUM
User Experience										
User interface										
Complexity										
Data entry ease										
Documentation										
External dependencies										
Performance										

SOURCE: Adapted from Aversano and Tortorella, 2004, p. 267.

NOTE: IM&T = Directorate of Information Management and Technology.

Stakeholders and Program Offices

List of Subject-Matter Experts

- GHE practitioners
  - AFRICOM Command Surgeon
  - Air Force Medical Readiness Agency
  - Air Force Special Operations Command (AFSOC)
  - Air Forces Southern (AFSOUTH)
  - CENTCOM
  - CENTCOM Command Surgeon
  - CGHE
  - CGHE Uniformed Services University of the Health Sciences
  - EUCOM Command Surgeon
  - INDOPACOM
  - INDOPACOM Center for Excellence in Disaster Management and Humanitarian Assistance
  - INDOPACOM Command Surgeon
  - National Guard Bureau
  - Navy Bureau of Medicine and Surgery
  - Pacific Air Forces (PACAF)
  - PACAF Command Surgeon
  - SOUTHCOM
  - SOUTHCOM Command Surgeon
  - SOCOM
  - Special Operations Command South (SOCSOUTH) Command Surgeon
  - U.S. Air Forces Central (AFCENT) Command Surgeon
  - U.S. Air Forces in Europe–Air Forces Africa (USAFE/AFAFRICA)
  - USAFE/AFAFRICA International Health Specialist Program
  - U.S. Army Medical Center of Excellence
  - U.S. Army Pacific (USARPAC)
  - U.S. Army Special Operations Command (USASOC) Command Surgeon
  - U.S. Army Veterinary Corps
  - U.S. Marine Corps Forces, Pacific (MARFORPAC) Office of the Force Surgeon
  - U.S. Pacific Fleet (PACFLT)
- Information system program offices
  - Advana
  - APAN (received only documentation)
  - Command and Control of the Information Environment (C2IE; received only documentation)
  - CFR

- CTIMS
- DSCA Directorate of Information Management and Technology
- G-TSCMIS (received only documentation)
- JLLIS
- MedCOP
- National Geospatial-Intelligence Agency (NGA) AFRICOM GIS System (AFRICOM Medical Engagements)
- NCMI
- OHASIS
- Socium
- Theater Engagement Dashboard (TED)

In total, we held discussions with 38 GHE practitioners and 22 information system program managers.

Additional Tools and Platforms Used by GHE

In this appendix, we describe the tools and platforms that support GHE in addition to those described in Chapter 4. In discussion with GHE stakeholders, we found these tools and platforms typically provide an important and targeted capability to GHE and the broader DoD community but are not tied to planning, request for funding, or tracking activities and engagements.

Table D.1 lists the platforms used by the GHE community and practitioners across GCCs. Many of the platforms, as described in Chapter 4, are homegrown or COTS platforms used exclusively for a specific type of funding (e.g., OHASIS) or exclusively by one or two GCCs and their component commands (e.g., CFR, CTIMS, and TED).

Additionally, for the GHE Intellipedia feasibility study, we spoke with NCMI representatives for architectural considerations for a platform for storing, accessing, and sharing intelligence.

TABLE D.1

Platforms for Tracking Activities and After-Action Reviews and for Analytics

Platform	Management	Used by GHE Practitioners
Advana	Under Secretary of Defense for Acquisition and Sustainment, DSCA	O
APAN	Office of the Administrative Assistant to the Secretary of the Air Force, INDOPACOM	O
C2IE	DSCA, Joint Staff	O
CFR	EUCOM, AFRICOM, CENTCOM	✓
CTIMS	SOUTHCOM	✓
G-TSCMIS	DSCA, combatant command	✓
GIS	NGA, AFRICOM	✓
Joint Civil Information Management System (JCIMS)	Joint Staff	X
JLLIS	OSD, Joint Staff	✓
MedCOP	EUCOM	O
OHASIS	DSCA, combatant command	✓
Socium	DSCA, combatant command	✓
Security Cooperation Information Portal	DSCA	X
TED	SOUTHCOM	✓

NOTE: Green (✓) = used by GHE practitioners for activity tracking; yellow (O) = used only for specific events, or platform is in development for specific needs, such as analytics; red (X) = no information from stakeholders or program offices.

Advana

Advana[1] is an analytics platform for enterprise-wide authoritative data management and analytics for OSD. It houses a collection of enterprise data as a data warehouse and supports decisionmaking across DoD and business with support analytics, visualizations, and various support services. Developed as an authoritative source for audit and business data analytics, Advana hosts more than 15 billion transactions, with more than 7,000 users and 250-plus dashboards as of 2020.[2] Advana has an automated data pipeline from more than 120 source systems from the broad DoD community and reconciles more than $1 trillion in financial transactions. It has the flexibility to support analytics in the areas of audit, financial operations, cost management, and performance management. As an example, it is used by the Defense Commissary Agency to automate quarterly review processes and expose funds at risk of expiring or canceling. Across OSD, Advana is used to improve data-sharing and transparency with a centralized repository of acquisition data.[3]

All Partners Access Network

APAN is an unclassified shared enterprise service dating back to 1997 that provides structured (via Share-Point) and unstructured (via Verint Telligent) collaboration capabilities with multinational partners, NGOs, and various U.S. federal and state agencies.[4] APAN also makes use of ESRI ArcGIS analytic and visualization capabilities. APAN is not inherently responsible for any data: All data sets are imported via other activity tracking and managing systems (most notably, OHASIS). Although the number of users and communities continues to increase every year (to approximately 224,000 users in 2018), the user turnover rate is significant, with 30.1 percent of users returning in 2018. Some examples of communities are typhoon support in the Philippines, disease outbreak in Africa, and earthquake support in Nepal.[5]

Verint Telligent

In 2010, APAN provided its users with the ability to create social media–like platforms (called groups) to collaborate in an unstructured manner using the Telligent platform provided by Verint (Figure D.1). Designed to be accessible and intuitive for nontechnical users, a group focuses on social engagements, and the main applications include blogs, discussion forums, media galleries, wikis, and calendars. Users can provide feedback at various levels of formality, from direct comments to tags, mentions, and likes.

SharePoint

Users looking for more-structured content can also create sites using SharePoint, which was added to APAN in 2013 (Figure D.2). Notable SharePoint capabilities include more-robust document and file management, calendars, event registration, and web conferencing.

---

[1]   The name Advana is derived from the phrase *advancing analytics* (Office of the Under Secretary of Defense (Comptroller), "Advana 2021 Strategy," 2021).

[2]   David L. Norquist, "Senate Armed Service Committee Subcommittee on Readiness Written Statement for the Record," November 20, 2019.

[3]   Office of the Under Secretary of Defense, Acquisition Analytics and Policy, October 13, 2021.

[4]   Verint, homepage, undated.

[5]   All Partners Access Network, "APAN Overview 2019: History, Governance, Capabilities, Use Cases, Statistics and POCs," 2019.

FIGURE D.1

Example APAN Telligent Platform

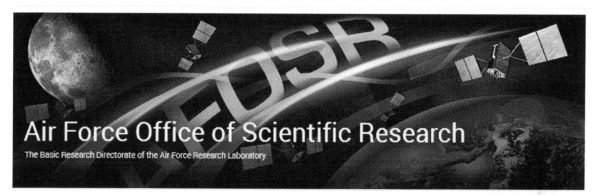

Air Force Office of Scientific Research

 — AFOSR

Research Areas   Events   Secure Upload   Public File Share   More

+ New

Air Force Office of Scientific Research
The Basic Research Directorate of the Air Force Research Laboratory

PRESENTATIONS DIRECTORY

Download presentations from past meetings and reviews at our presentations directory.

- Research Areas
  - Aerospace Materials for Extreme Environments
  - Aerothermodynamics
  - Atomic and Molecular Physics
  - Biophysics
  - Complex Network Systems
  - Computational Cognition and Machine Intelligence
  - Computational Mathematics
  - Dynamic Data Driven Applications Systems (DDDAS)
  - Dynamic Materials and Interactions
  - Dynamics and Control
  - Electromagnetics

BASIC RESEARCH FUNDING OPPORTUNITIES

AFOSR invites proposals in broad research areas through the general BAA and other broad agency announcements. Proposals submitted under the BAAs are evaluated using a peer or scientific review process and selected for award on a competitive basis.

To apply for AFOSR funding opportunities listed in the BAA, visit www.grants.gov. All application forms and instructions are provided on the site. You can search grants.gov by CDFA numbers 12.800, 12.630 and 12.910. There you can also search for opportunities by all grant issuing agencies.

Quick Links:
2015 AFOSR BAA
AFOSR Funding Opportunities
Search for other opportunities on Grants.gov

WELCOME

We're excited to use APAN to effectively communicate and collaborate with researchers around the world.

GET STARTED
In order to use all of the features APAN provides, you'll need to take two quick steps.

1. Become a member of APAN
2. Join the AFOSR group

STAY CONNECTED

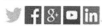

Technical Strategic Plan

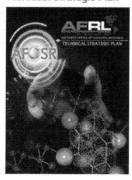

Download the Technical Strategic Plan

Did you know?

Did you know that as of 2014, AFOSR basic research funding had resulted in or contributed to

SOURCE: Reproduced from APAN, 2019.

FIGURE D.2
Example APAN SharePoint Platform

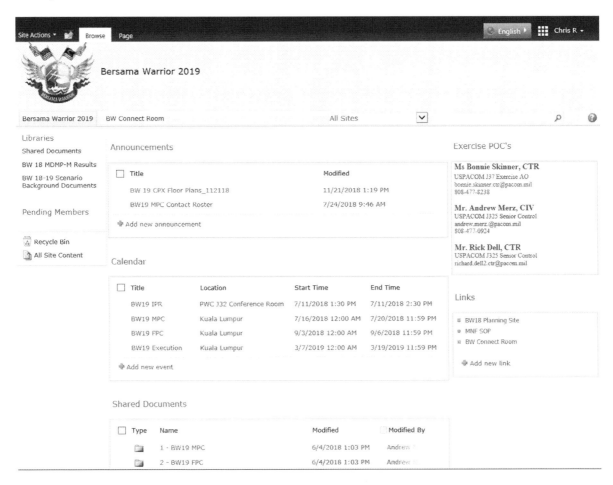

SOURCE: Reproduced from APAN, 2019.

Command and Control of the Information Environment

C2IE provides an integrated view of joint force plans and orders; U.S. military operations, activities, and investments; and U.S. partner nations, government and military, and competition intelligence. C2IE, therefore, is an integrated information exchange platform. It provides data analytics capability with AI integration. C2IE is being used by the joint force to support the GCCs and joint force operations. C2IE use for data analytics was being independently considered for GHE support by some GCCs at the time of our study. The platform was scheduled to have a one-way data-pull integration with Socium in FY 2021. However, GHE planners do not see C2IE as a long-term solution for data analytics or advanced analytics support.

Cloud-Based TCA Information Management System

CTIMS is the authoritative data source for all TCA-funded operations, activities, and investments within SOUTHCOM. Events include conferences, seminars, SME exchanges, key leader engagements, orientations, assessments, and schoolhouse visits designed to encourage a democratic orientation of defense establishments and security forces of other countries. Historically, CTIMS acts as the local repository; activity data are later duplicated on the G-TSCMIS system and interface with the TED platform.[6]

NGA-AFRICOM GIS (AFRICOM Medical Engagements)

The AFRICOM Command Surgeon's office uses NGA-AFRICOM GIS to track, analyze, and visualize its medical engagements in the AOR. AFRICOM GIS provides event creation and monitoring, area-wide activity mapping, and reporting capabilities.[7] AFRICOM GIS has been effective for the GHE monthly working group when used in conjunction with data provided by CFR and OHASIS.[8] Similar capabilities either exist or are being developed on both the Socium and MedCOP platforms.[9]

Joint Civil Information Management System

JCIMS is maintained by the Maritime Civil Affairs and Security Training Command. JCIMS provides information on civil affairs (such as infrastructure and medical capabilities) and civil-military operations in a collaborative environment. JCIMS is focused on identifying the joint tactics, techniques, and procedures for a standardized process for the collection, consolidation, and sharing of civil information across multiple environments.

Theater Engagement Dashboard

TED is an IT platform available on the NIPR and SIPR systems that compiles security cooperation activities data from CTIMS, OHASIS, and G-TSCMIS. TED NIPR is authorized for up to UNCLASSIFIED//FOR OFFICIAL USE ONLY information and requires a CAC to gain access, and all accounts are reviewed and approved with the J54 (Strategic Plans Division). TED assists in the planning process with calendar visualizations and country- or agency-specific libraries for SSCI, and other relevant documents. TED also has the ability to create joint operations, activities, and investments. Since the transition to Socium, TED was transitioned to read-only in summer 2021.

---

[6] Potomac Officers Club, "USSOUTHCOM Seeks IT Services for Engagement Event Tracker," December 27, 2021; and Standard Operating Procedure 2000.01, State Partnership Program (SOP), Texas Military Department, January 1, 2019.

[7] Product demonstration, November 2020.

[8] Conversations with AFRICOM Geospatial Intelligence Support, 2020.

[9] Conversations with Socium and MedCOP program management, 2020–2021.

Abbreviations

AAR	after-action review
AFRICOM	U.S. Africa Command
AI	artificial intelligence
AIDE	Automated Information Discovery Environment
AM&E	assessment, monitoring, and evaluation
AOR	area of responsibility
APAN	All Partners Access Network
C2IE	Command and Control of the Information Environment (data analytics platform)
CAC	Common Access Card
CBA	capabilities-based assessment
CENTCOM	U.S. Central Command
CFR	Concept and Funding Request
CGHE	Center for Global Health Engagement
COP	common operating picture
COTS	commercial off-the shelf
COVID-19	coronavirus disease 2019
CTIMS	Cloud-Based TCA Information Management System
DCR	DOTmLPF-P Change Recommendation
DHA	Defense Health Agency
DIA	Defense Intelligence Agency
DoD	U.S. Department of Defense
DOTmLPF-P	Doctrine, Organization, Training, materiel, Leadership and education, Personnel, Facilities, and Policy
DSCA	Defense Security Cooperation Agency
EUCOM	U.S. European Command
FY	fiscal year
G-TSCMIS	Global-Theater Security Cooperation Management Information System
GCC	geographic combatant command

GHE	global health engagement
GIS	Geographic Information System
INDOPACOM	U.S. Indo-Pacific Command
IPT	Integrated Product Team
IT	information technology
JCIMS	Joint Civil Information Management System
JLLIS	Joint Lessons Learned Information System
JLLP	Joint Lessons Learned Process
JOMIS	Joint Operational Medicine Information System
JWICS	Joint Worldwide Intelligence Communication System
MedCOP	Medical Common Operating Picture
NCMI	National Center for Medical Intelligence
NGA	National Geospatial-Intelligence Agency
NGO	nongovernmental organization
NIPR	Non-classified Internet Protocol Router
OASD(HA)	Office of the Assistant Secretary of Defense for Health Affairs
OHASIS	Overseas Humanitarian Assistance Shared Information System
OHDACA	Overseas Humanitarian, Disaster, and Civic Aid
OSD	Office of the Secretary of Defense
SAAR	System Authorization Access Request
SIPR	Secret Internet Protocol Router
SMART	Specific, Measurable, Achievable, Realistic, and Time-bound
SME	subject-matter expert
SOCOM	U.S. Special Operations Command
SOUTHCOM	U.S. Southern Command
SSCI	Significant Security Cooperation Initiative
TCA	Traditional Combatant Command Activities
TCP	Theater Campaign Plan
TED	Theater Engagement Dashboard
TSCMIS	Theater Security Cooperation Management Information System

References

All Partners Access Network, "APAN Overview 2019: History, Governance, Capabilities, Use Cases, Statistics and POCs," 2019.

Aversano, Lerina, and Maria Tortorella, "An Assessment Strategy for Identifying Legacy System Evolution Requirements in eBusiness Context," *Journal of Software Maintenance and Evolution: Research and Practice*, Vol. 16, No. 4–5, July–October 2004.

Ayotte, Kelly, Julie Gerberding, and J. Stephen Morrison, *Ending the Cycle of Crisis and Complacency in U.S. Global Health Security. A Report of the CSIS Commission on Strengthening America's Health Security*, Center for Strategic and International Studies, November 2019.

Chairman of the Joint Chiefs of Staff Instruction 3150.25H, *Joint Lessons Learned Program*, Joint Chiefs of Staff, December 30, 2021.

Chairman of the Joint Chiefs of Staff Instruction 5123.01H, *Charter of the Joint Requirements Oversight Council (JROC) and Implementation of the Joint Capabilities Integration and Development System (JCIDS)*, Joint Chiefs of Staff, August 31, 2018.

Chairman of the Joint Chiefs of Staff Manual 3150.25B, *Joint Lessons Learned Program*, Joint Chiefs of Staff, October 12, 2018.

Connor, Kathryn, Ian P. Cook, Isaac R. Porche III, and Daniel Gonzales, *Cost Considerations in Cloud Computing*, RAND Corporation, PE-113-A, 2014. As of January 5, 2023:
https://www.rand.org/pubs/perspectives/PE113.html

Crotty, James, and Ivan Horrocks, "Managing Legacy System Costs: A Case Study of a Meta-Assessment Model to Identify Solutions in a Large Financial Services Company," *Applied Computing and Informatics*, Vol. 13, No. 2, July 2017.

Defense Healthcare Management Systems, "Joint Operational Medicine Information Systems," fact sheet, July 2020.

Defense Security Cooperation Agency, "Socium—Building a Security Cooperation Management System Overview," briefing, 2020a, Not available to the general public.

Defense Security Cooperation Agency, "DSCA Socium SAAR Guide," provided to the authors by Socium Program Management, December 2020b, Not available to the general public.

Defense Security Cooperation Agency, *Department of Defense Fiscal Year (FY) 2022 Budget Estimates: Research, Development, Test & Evaluation, Defense-Wide*, May 2021a.

Defense Security Cooperation Agency, *Fiscal Year 2022 President's Budget: Operation and Maintenance, Defense-Wide*, May 2021b.

Defense Security Cooperation Agency, Institute of Security Governance, "Institutional Capacity Building: An Essential Component of Full Spectrum Capability Development," January 2021.

Defense Security Cooperation Agency IT Program Management, "Socium System Interfaces," February 2021, Not available to the general public.

DeFilippi, Gwendolyn R., Stephen Francis Nowak, and Bradford Harlow Baylor, "The Importance of Lessons Learned in Joint Force Development," *Joint Force Quarterly*, No. 89, April 2018.

Department of Defense Directive 5132.03, *DoD Policy and Responsibilities Relating to Security Cooperation*, U.S. Department of Defense, December 29, 2016.

Department of Defense Instruction 2000.30, *Global Health Engagement (GHE) Activities*, U.S. Department of Defense, July 12, 2017. As of March 28, 2021:
https://www.esd.whs.mil/Portals/54/Documents/DD/issuances/dodi/200030_dodi_2017.pdf

Department of Defense Instruction 5132.14, *Assessment, Monitoring, and Evaluation Policy for the Security Cooperation Enterprise*, U.S. Department of Defense, January 13, 2017.

DeSitter, Betsy, and Max Ramirez, "MedCOP: A Step Towards Purple," *Medical Leader*, blog, October 22, 2020. As of July 25, 2022:
https://medium.com/experientia-et-progressus/medcop-a-step-towards-purple-eeba07c0345

DoD—*See* U.S. Department of Defense.

Grill, Beth, Trupti Brahmbhatt, Pauline Moore, Jennifer D. P. Moroney, and Chandler Sachs, *Funding Global Health Engagement to Support the Geographic Combatant Commands*, RAND Corporation, RR-A1357-2, 2023. As of June 2023:
https://www.rand.org/pubs/research_reports/RRA1357-2.html

Grill, Beth, Michael J. McNerney, Jeremy Boback, Renanah Miles, Cynthia C. Clapp-Wincek, and David E. Thaler, *Follow the Money: Promoting Greater Transparency in Department of Defense Security Cooperation Reporting*, RAND Corporation, RR-2039-OSD, 2017. As of January 5, 2023:
https://www.rand.org/pubs/research_reports/RR2039.html

Joint Publication 3-20, *Security Cooperation*, Joint Chiefs of Staff, May 23, 2017. As of November 14, 2022:
https://www.jcs.mil/Portals/36/Documents/Doctrine/pubs/jp3_20_20172305.pdf

Joint Publication 3-29, *Foreign Humanitarian Assistance*, Joint Chiefs of Staff, May 14, 2019. As of April 27, 2022:
https://www.jcs.mil/Portals/36/Documents/Doctrine/pubs/jp3_29.pdf

Leclerc-Madlala, Suzanne, and Maysaa Alobaidi, "Sharpening Our Cultural Tools for Improved Global Health Engagement," *Joint Force Quarterly*, No. 82, July 2016.

Marquis, Jefferson P., Trupti Brahmbhatt, Aaron Clark-Ginsberg, Victoria M. Smith, and David E. Thaler, *Educating and Training the Department of Defense Workforce for Global Health Engagement to Support the Geographic Combatant Commands*, RAND Corporation, RR-A1357-1, 2023. As of June 2023:
https://www.rand.org/pubs/research_reports/RRA1357-1.html

Marquis, Jefferson P., David E. Thaler, S. Rebecca Zimmerman, Megan Stewart, and Jeremy Boback, *The Global-Theater Security Cooperation Management Information System: Assessment and Implications for Strategic Users*, RAND Corporation, RR-1680-OSD, 2016, Not available to the general public.

Marquis, Jefferson P., Richard E. Darilek, Jasen J. Castillo, Cathryn Quantic Thurston, Anny Wong, Cynthia Huger, Andrea Mejia, Jennifer D. P. Moroney, Brian Nichiporuk, and Brett Steele, *Assessing the Value of U.S. Army International Activities*, RAND Corporation, MG-329-A, 2006. As of January 5, 2023:
https://www.rand.org/pubs/monographs/MG329.html

McNerney, Michael J., Jefferson P. Marquis, S. Rebecca Zimmerman, and Ariel Klein, *SMART Security Cooperation Objectives: Improving DoD Planning and Guidance*, RAND Corporation, RR-1430-OSD, 2016. As of January 5, 2023:
https://www.rand.org/pubs/research_reports/RR1430.html

MediaWiki, homepage, undated. As of July 25, 2022:
https://www.mediawiki.org/wiki/MediaWiki

Mendez, Bryce H. P., Sara M. Tharakan, and Emily K. Lane, "Department of Defense Global Health Engagement," Congressional Research Service, IF11386, updated January 16, 2020.

Norquist, David L., "Senate Armed Service Committee Subcommittee on Readiness Written Statement for the Record," November 20, 2019.

Novetta, "AIDE: Automated Information Discovery Environment," fact sheet, September 22, 2021. As of February 10, 2022:
https://www.novetta.com/2021/09/aide/

Office of the Under Secretary of Defense, Acquisition Analytics and Policy, October 13, 2021.

Office of the Under Secretary of Defense (Comptroller), "Advana 2021 Strategy," 2021.

O'Mahony, Angela, Ilana Blum, Gabriela Armenta, Nicholas E. Burger, Joshua Mendelsohn, Michael J. McNerney, Steven W. Popper, Jefferson P. Marquis, and Thomas S. Szayna, *Assessing, Monitoring, and Evaluating Army Security Cooperation: A Framework for Implementation*, RAND Corporation, RR-2165-A, 2018. As of January 5, 2023:
https://www.rand.org/pubs/research_reports/RR2165.html

Perry, Walter L., Stuart Johnson, Stephanie Pezard, Gillian S. Oak, David Stebbins, and Chaoling Feng, *Defense Institution Building: An Assessment*, RAND Corporation, RR-1176-OSD, 2016. As of January 5, 2023: https://www.rand.org/pubs/research_reports/RR1176.html

Potomac Officers Club, "USSOUTHCOM Seeks IT Services for Engagement Event Tracker," December 27, 2021. As of February 12, 2022: https://potomacofficersclub.com/news/ussouthcom-seeks-it-services-for-engagement-event-tracker/

Ransom, Jane, Ian Sommerville, and Ian Warren, "A Method for Assessing Legacy Systems for Evolution," *Proceedings of the Second Euromicro Conference on Software Maintenance and Reengineering*, 1998.

Seacord, Robert C., Daniel Plakosh, and Grace A. Lewis, *Modernizing Legacy Systems: Software Technologies, Engineering Processes, and Business Practices*, Addison-Wesley, 2003.

Selva, Paul, Vice Chairman of the Joint Chiefs of Staff, "DOTmLPF-P Change Recommendation for Global Health Engagement," memorandum, JROCM 008-19, February 25, 2019, Not available to the general public.

Sherman, John B., U.S. Department of Defense Chief Information Officer, "Software Development and Open Source Software," memorandum for senior Pentagon leadership, Commandant of the Coast Guard, commanders of the combatant commands, and defense agency and DoD field activity directors, January 24, 2022.

Shoreland Travax, homepage, undated. As of April 15, 2021: https://www.travax.com/

Sledge, Carol, and David Carney, "Case Study: Evaluating COTS Products for DoD Information Systems," Software Engineering Institute, Carnegie Mellon University, June 1998.

Socium Program Management, "Socium Monthly Demonstration," Defense Security Cooperation Agency, December 2020 to January 2022.

Standard Operating Procedure 2000.01, *State Partnership Program (SPP)*, Texas Military Department, January 1, 2019. As of January 5, 2023: https://tmd.texas.gov/Data/Sites/1/media/tmdpolicies/publications/tmd-sop-2000_01-state-partnership-program-spp-dated.pdf

Treverton, Gregory F., *New Tools for Collaboration: The Experience of the U.S. Intelligence Community*, Center for Strategic and International Studies, January 2016.

Tripathy, Priyadarshi, and Kshirasagar Naik, *Software Evolution and Maintenance: A Practitioner's Approach*, Wiley, 2015.

Uniformed Services University, "Department of Defense Global Health Engagement," briefing, undated, Not available to the general public.

U.S. Code, Title 10, Section 333, Foreign Security Forces: Authority to Build Capacity.

U.S. Code, Title 10, Section 345, Regional Defense Combating Terrorism and Irregular Warfare Fellowship Program.

U.S. Department of Defense, *Global Health Engagement (GHE) Capabilities-Based Assessment (CBA) Study*, July 23, 2018, Not available to the general public.

U.S. Department of Defense, Military Health System, "Global Health Engagement," webpage, undated. As of January 20, 2022: https://www.health.mil/Military-Health-Topics/Health-Readiness/Global-Health-Engagement

U.S. European Command J5/8 Security Cooperation and Partnering Division, *M2M and Concept & Funding Request (CFR) User Guide*, May 20, 2020.

U.S. Southern Command, "Global Health Engagement Strengthens Partnerships," January 6, 2020. As of November 1, 2021: https://www.southcom.mil/MEDIA/NEWS-ARTICLES/Article/2050739/global-health-engagement-strengthens-partnerships/

Verint, homepage, undated. As of January 5, 2023: https://www.verint.com

Wissemann, Michael W., "Great (Soft) Power Competition: US and Chinese Efforts in Global Health Engagement," *Parameters*, Vol. 51, No. 3, August 2021.